THE
PSYCHEDELIC
REAWAKENING

"A well-researched, up-to-date summary of what's on the cutting edge of the psychedelic renaissance, covering the latest neuroscience, clinical trials, and therapeutic potential of psychedelic medicines. *The Psychedelic Reawakening* is a crash course in psychoactive drugs, a wonderful overview of some of the most promising and powerful tools for treating mental health, and a valuable guide to learning harm reduction strategies. After so many years of psychedelics being criminalized, demonized, ridiculed, or ignored, Anton Gomez-Escolar's *The Psychedelic Reawakening* is a breath of fresh air!"

DAVID JAY BROWN, AUTHOR OF
THE ILLUSTRATED FIELD GUIDE TO DMT ENTITIES AND
THE NEW SCIENCE OF PSYCHEDELICS

"Gomez-Escolar expands our view of the vast potential of psychedelics for therapeutic use. He emphasizes that the use of such substances requires purposeful intention through set and setting to maximize benefits and promote safe use. *The Psychedelic Reawakening* is an excellent resource for therapists and other health professionals and their clients, policy makers, recreational users, psychonauts, and the general public."

WADE RICHARDSON, AUTHOR OF
THE PSYCHEDELIC MINDMELD

"*The Psychedelic Reawakening* is relevant and necessary at a time when psychedelic drugs are already available for use in psychiatry, as is the case with ketamine, and as the available arsenal will grow over time: psilocybin, MDMA, DMT, and more. This book fills a necessary gap in this new medical and social panorama. In addition, Anton Gomez-Escolar is one of the best specialists in this field in Spain. *The Psychedelic Reawakening* will also serve to provide the media with objective and accessible information on a subject that, although still unknown, will be the future of mental health treatment, at a time when it is more necessary than ever."

JOSÉ CARLOS BOUSO, PH.D., SCIENTIFIC DIRECTOR OF
THE INTERNATIONAL CENTER FOR
ETHNOBOTANICAL EDUCATION,
RESEARCH, AND SERVICE

THE

PSYCHEDELIC REAWAKENING

How Psilocybin,
MDMA, Ketamine, LSD, and DMT
Are Changing Lives

Anton Gomez-Escolar,
MSc, MPH, MIR

Park Street Press
Rochester, Vermont

Park Street Press
One Park Street
Rochester, Vermont 05767
www.ParkStPress.com

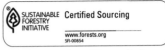

Text stock is SFI certified

Park Street Press is a division of Inner Traditions International

Originally published in 2022 as *Essential Guide to the Psychedelic Renaissance* by
Argonowta Digital SSL, Madrid, Spain

*Note to the Reader: This book is intended as an informational guide and should not be a
substitute for professional medical care or treatment. Neither the author nor the publisher
assumes any responsibility for physical, psychological, legal, or social consequences resulting
from the ingestion of psychedelic substances or their derivatives.*

Cataloging-in-Publication Data for this title is available from the Library of Congress

ISBN 979-8-88850-002-6 (print)
ISBN 979-8-88850-003-3 (ebook)

Printed and bound in the United States by Lake Book Manufacturing, LLC
The text stock is SFI certified. The Sustainable Forestry Initiative® program promotes
sustainable forest management.

10 9 8 7 6 5 4 3 2 1

Text design by Virginia Bowmen and layout by Kenleigh Manseau
This book was typeset in Garamond Premier Pro with Nexa used as a display font

Creative Commons Agreements: CC0: pg. 188; CC BY 2.0: pg. 92; CC BY-SA 2.0: pg. 22,
pg. 54; CC BY-SA 2.0 DE: pg. 80; CC BY-SA 2.5: pg. 174, plate 20; CC BY 3.0: pg. 3,
pg. 160, pg. 166, pg. 170, plate 17, plate 19; CC BY-SA 3.0: pg. 4, pg. 9, pg. 14, pg. 24,
pg. 25, pg. 39, pg. 82, pg. 148, pg. 154, pg. 169, pg. 256, plate 1, plate 14, plate 15, plate 18,
plate 25; CC BY 4.0: pg. 8, pg. 106, pg. 327, plate 2, plate 10; CC BY-SA 4.0: pg. 2, pg. 31,
pg. 34, pg. 86, pg. 119, pg. 158, pg. 161, pg. 175, pg. 180, pg. 261, pg. 267, plate 16, plate 21.

To send correspondence to the author of this book, mail a first-class letter to the author c/o
Inner Traditions • Bear & Company, One Park Street, Rochester, VT 05767, and we will
forward the communication, or contact the author directly at **antongomezes.com**.

Scan the QR code and save 25% at InnerTraditions.com.
Browse over 2,000 titles on spirituality, the occult, ancient
mysteries, new science, holistic health, and natural medicine.

To so many brave and unprejudiced people,
who prefer to listen and research before speaking,
who question dogmas and make the world move forward.

To family and good friends,
to love and other miracles of life.
Thank you for always being there for me.

Contents

FOREWORD
by Rick Doblin, Ph.D. xi

Preface xv

1 Basic Concepts of Neuroscience and
   Neuropharmacology 1
   The Brain and Central Nervous System 1
   Neurons, Synapses, Neurotransmitters, and
       Neuroreceptors 3
   Neuropharmacology 9

2 Introduction to Psychoactive Substances 12
   Talking about Psychoactive Substances 12
   Types of Psychoactive Substances 14
   Stimulants 18
   Depressants 20
   Opioids 23
   Cannabinoids 24
   Empathogens/Entactogens 26
   Dissociatives 30
   Psychedelics 33

3 A History of Psychedelics in the West 38
   Pre-LSD 38
   Post-LSD 40
   MDMA 63
   After the Ban 67

4 The Psychedelic Renaissance   **71**

Ongoing Psychedelics Research   73
Social and Cultural Contexts   87
The Rise of a New Industry   93

5 How Psychedelics Work   **98**

Mechanisms at the Neuroreceptor Level   98
Mechanisms at the Brain Level   100
How Does the Brain Work? Hierarchical Predictive Coding   101
How Do Psychedelics Affect Our Brain Function?   105
What Happens at the Psychological Level?   108
Why Do We Have 5-HT2a Receptors and
    Psychedelic Experiences?   111
How Can Psychedelics Help with Mental Health
    Disorders or Other Maladaptive Conditions?   112

**6 The Present and Future of Clinical Research
with Psychedelic Drugs**   **116**

Psychedelic-Assisted Psychotherapy   116
Post-Traumatic Stress Disorder (PTSD)   119
Depression and Anxiety   125
Addictions   134
Neurodegenerative Diseases, Long COVID,
    and Neurorehabiliation   140
Behavior Change   142
Couples Therapy and Conflict Resolution   142
Microdosing   143
Other Lines of Research for Possible Future Applications   145

**7 The Applications, Effects, Dosages, and
Risks of Different Psychedelic Substances**   **146**

Psilocybin ("Magic Mushrooms")   146
LSD ("Acid")   153
DMT/Ayahuasca   158
5-MeO-DMT ("Toad")   164
Mescaline ("Cactus")   167
Ibogaine   173
MDMA ("Ecstasy")   177
Ketamine   186

8 Psychedelic Risks and Harm Reduction Strategies   192

Risks Related to Substance (Drug)   198
Dosage, Frequency of Consumption, and Tolerance   198
Purity and Adulteration   201
Routes of Administration   205
Mixtures and Combinations   207
Risks Related to Person and Context (Set and Setting)   208
Minimizing Risks Related to the Set   209
Minimizing Risks Related to the Setting   211
Managing "Bad Trips" and other Psychedelic Emergencies   213

9 Conclusions: Looking to the Future   217

APPENDIX I
Psychedelic Resources   225

APPENDIX II
**The Legal Status of Psychedelic Drugs
around the World   234**

APPENDIX III
Glossary   271

Index   280

Foreword

Rick Doblin, Ph.D.

In the 1970s and '80s, most psychedelic substances as well as psychedelic research were banned nationally and internationally, despite millennia of traditional use, decades of western scientific studies, and neuroscience discoveries and promising results in mental health treatments (as you will learn in this book). The western sociopolitical context then was different from today's, with limited social and scientific knowledge about these powerful substances. There was little in the way of accurate harm reduction information to effectively minimize the risks of the widespread recreational use, and the clinical use was blocked by the massive "war on drugs" propaganda so as not to counteract the misinformation. Psychedelics were lacking more solid scientific knowledge and, as humans, we tend to fear what we don't fully know, control, or understand, so psychedelics were brought to a difficult impasse. In 1986, to break that impasse with new scientific research and knowledge, right after the 1985 scheduling of MDMA (3,4-methylenedioxymethamphetamine), I founded the scientific research and educational nonprofit MAPS (the Multidisciplinary Association for Psychedelic Studies), which develops medical, legal, and cultural contexts for people to benefit from the careful uses of psychedelics.

For more than thirty years, despite all the difficulties, the knowledge about these powerful tools was kept and expanded both underground and beginning in 2000 in clinical research into therapeutic applications, thanks to the conviction of many brave therapists, activists, scientists, and organizations like MAPS, convinced that psychedelics were "as valuable to the mind as the telescope is to astronomy or the microscope is to biology" (to cite Stanislav Grof) and hold immense therapeutic potential. With the new millennia, the research started giving us its fruits, and all this important scientific wisdom started to appear in modern science here and there in the context of the big mental health epidemic unfolding in the western societies over the last decades, an epidemic that current mental health treatments are struggling unsuccessfully to contain. The enormous potential of psychedelics for neuroscience and therapy attracted the interest of many great scientists and institutions worldwide who joined the field and further accelerated the research and the momentum for accepted medical use.

Nowadays, in the midst of a psychedelic renaissance with the potential to transform mental health treatments and our knowledge of the mind forever, esketamine has already been approved for treating depression since 2019. Also, phase 3 trials[1] with MDMA-assisted therapy for treatment-resistant post-traumatic stress disorder (PTSD) provided great results that point to a future authorization of this therapy in the U.S. and the E.U. in the next few years, while psilocybin and other psychedelic compounds are researched for many different mental health indications and might follow. Since 2023 Australia has already authorized some licensed psychiatrists to use both MDMA and psilocybin to treat treatment-resistant PTSD and depression, respectively. We have more and more psychedelic knowledge every day. We also have a great opportunity to make all this new scientific knowledge accessible for everyone, to make people understand how and why psychedelic-assisted therapies work, and why all this scientific research is good news for public health. We can finally bring these treatments to those who need them in a context where society understands what, why, and how. This is the aim of this book.

---

1. A phase 3 clinical trial is a large-scale study that tests the efficacy and monitors the adverse reactions of a new treatment or drug in diverse patient populations to confirm its safety and effectiveness before regulatory approval.

In this this book, you will learn about the basics of psychedelic drugs, the history of the psychedelic renaissance, the new neuroscience discoveries made through psychedelics, and the very promising uses of psychedelic-assisted psychotherapies to treat many difficult indications like depression, anxiety, PTSD, and addiction. You will also learn about the potential risks and practical harm reduction approaches used to prevent these risks inside and outside the lab. Psychedelic substances are now in the process of demonstrating safety and efficacy because we now know more about how to better manage the variables of set and setting to maximize possibilities of a therapeutic outcome and minimize the risk of any problem when psychedelics are taken in a proper therapeutic context with a proper mindset and preparation.

Knowledge is power. To make this psychedelic revolution become an enduring clinical reality for millions of patients and humanity, we need our societies to be well educated in the topic to avoid past mistakes and to understand the potential risks and benefits, avoiding the former and benefiting from the latter, like many other cultures around the world have done for millennia. After decades of propaganda and misinformation, a well-informed public opinion through books like this one is the safe way forward for science, public health, and to counteract the prohibitionist approaches to drugs we still face in many places. Despite the amazing results and safety shown for psychedelics in the clinical studies so far, a lot of understanding, work, and legal developments are still needed in most countries and societies to keep researching, optimizing, and finally bringing these powerful tools to those who need them now for therapy and those who might benefit from them in the future. We need good public and administrative knowledge for more research and to set the basis for an informed debate on how to better utilize the amazing opportunities brought to us by the psychedelic renaissance.

An enduring legacy of the COVID-19 pandemic was an aggravated mental health epidemic requiring better therapeutic tools to cope with it, rising awareness about the importance of safe and effective mental health prevention and treatments, and the importance of trusting science. As you will read in these pages, science is showing that psychedelics are a powerful tool for mental health treatment and psychedelic-assisted psychotherapy is needed more than ever. Psychedelic research has the potential to change our approach to mental health forever, if we manage to keep educating society and minimizing risky use. After a very long and strange trip, psychedelics are finally back to stay.

RICK DOBLIN, PH.D.,
FOUNDER AND PRESIDENT OF MAPS

RICK DOBLIN, PH.D., is the founder and president of the Multidisciplinary Association for Psychedelic Studies (MAPS). He received his doctorate in public policy from Harvard's Kennedy School of Government, where he wrote his dissertation on the regulation of the medical uses of psychedelics and marijuana and his master's thesis on a survey of oncologists about smoked marijuana versus the oral THC pill in nausea control for cancer patients. His undergraduate thesis at New College of Florida was a twenty-five-year follow-up to the classic Good Friday Experiment, which evaluated the potential of psychedelic drugs to catalyze religious experiences. He also conducted a thirty-four-year follow-up study to Timothy Leary's Concord Prison Experiment. Rick studied with Dr. Stanislav Grof and was among the first to be certified as a Holotropic Breathwork practitioner. His professional goal is to help develop legal contexts for the beneficial uses of psychedelics and marijuana, primarily as prescription medicines but also for personal growth for otherwise healthy people, and eventually to become a legally licensed psychedelic therapist. He founded MAPS in 1986, and currently resides in Boston with his wife and puppy, with three empty rooms from his children who have all graduated college and begun their life journeys. Learn more about Rick by listening to his Origin Story and watching his TED Talk.

Preface

This book will allow you to learn many things about psychoactive substances in general and psychedelics in particular, as well as the current status of their promising therapeutic uses for a variety of mental health disorders that are widespread today, unfortunately.

Providing a closer look at these issues, in a simple and instructive way, this book seeks to bring the subject within reach of anyone with an interest in psychedelics without neglecting scientific rigor and objectivity. I will avoid delving into moral or philosophical questions and instead focus on science, rational knowledge, pragmatism, and public health.

In this volume, I will begin by introducing the topic of psychoactive drugs, providing the reader with a basic understanding of their types, mechanisms of action, uses, and risks. I will then focus on the specific topic of psychedelic drugs—their recent history, their mechanisms of action, the growing scientific and clinical interest in psychedelics, their legal status, and how to reduce their risks as much as possible.

As you will discover in these pages, society is primed to learn about these issues. Not only are there growing movements clamoring for the failure of the "war on drugs" and calling for a revision of the policies in this regard (mainly aimed at drug decriminalization and even regulation), but there is an important research current that proposes the therapeutic use of some of these psychoactive substances, particularly cannabis (a compound which we will not focus on in great detail) and those with psychedelic properties, since they can become very effective treatments for some of the most difficult disorders we face in mental health today. These substances can be both classic psychedelics (psilocybin, LSD, mescaline, or ayahuasca) and empathogenic/entactogenic psychedelics (MDMA) or dissociative psychedelics (ketamine).[1]

Disorders such as depression, anxiety, addictions, or post-traumatic stress—widespread in modern Western societies and very difficult to treat successfully or efficiently—are being treated experimentally, even achieving complete remissions[2] in a safe and effective manner through the use of psychotherapies assisted by psychedelic (or semipsychedelic[3]) substances in controlled therapeutic contexts. These results have earned recognition from the most important regulatory agencies in the world, such as the U.S. Food and Drug Administration (FDA) and the European Union's EMA (European Medicines Agency), designating psychedelic-assisted psychotherapies with the designation of "breakthrough therapy" for having great innovative importance, to facilitate their research, and to accelerate their clinical development.

The return of these substances, which, decades ago—and in a very different sociopolitical context—were classified internationally as having "a high potential for abuse and no recognized medical value," a classification which led to their prohibition for most uses, means that we are now rediscovering these powerful molecules that have been used for millennia by many other cultures outside the Western world. For us, this means a real psychedelic reawakening, or as it's commonly referred, a *psychedelic renaissance*, the beginning of a revolution in neuroscience and mental health that could change our societies forever.

---

1. All of these substances are defined in chapter 2.
2. In mental health, the word "cure" is not used much; rather the concept of complete or partial "remission" is preferred.
3. Substances with psychedelic properties, even if these are not their main effect; also known as atypical psychedelics.

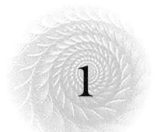

1

Basic Concepts of Neuroscience and Neuropharmacology

Before addressing issues of psychoactive drugs in general and those with psychedelic properties in particular, it is necessary to be clear about some basic concepts of neuroscience[1] that will allow us to understand both drugs' and specifically psychedelics' basic mechanisms of action and the elementary terminology necessary to be able to speak about them properly. In addition, you can find some key definitions in the glossary. Let's start by briefly exploring the terrain.

THE BRAIN AND CENTRAL NERVOUS SYSTEM

In the human body, our thoughts, emotions, and behaviors originate in the most complex and mysterious organ we have: the brain.

This organ is located inside our head and is part of what is known as the nervous system, a system that runs throughout our body and performs numerous functions for our survival, such as regulating and maintaining each vital function, controlling voluntary movements,

---

1. Science that studies the nervous system and all its aspects (such as structure, function, biochemistry, pharmacology and pathology), and how its different elements interact, giving rise to the biological bases of cognition and behavior.

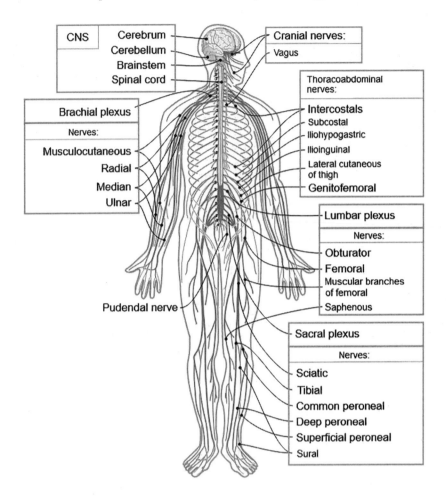

| CNS | Cerebrum |
| Cerebellum |
| Brainstem |
| Spinal cord |

Cranial nerves:
Vagus

Thoracoabdominal nerves:
Intercostals
Subcostal
Iliohypogastric
Ilioinguinal
Lateral cutaneous of thigh
Genitofemoral

Brachial plexus
Nerves:
Musculocutaneous
Radial
Median
Ulnar

Lumbar plexus
Nerves:
Obturator
Femoral
Muscular branches of femoral
Saphenous

Pudendal nerve

Sacral plexus
Nerves:
Sciatic
Tibial
Common peroneal
Deep peroneal
Superficial peroneal
Sural

Arrangement of the parts of the nervous system
(both central and peripheral) in the human body.
Image by Medium69, Jmarchn.

speech, intelligence, memory, emotions, and processing the information received through the senses. It is the organ where the mind and consciousness of the individual reside.

The brain is the directing part of this complex nerve network that extends throughout the body and allows it to carry out its important functions. Based on these functions and the anatomical structure, human beings divide our nervous system into the central nervous system, or CNS (which includes the brain and spinal cord), and the peripheral nervous system, or PNS (consisting of all the peripheral nerves that are outside the CNS but connect to it).

Both the central nervous system and the peripheral nervous system are made up of many different elements and subunits, but the most famous and important are highly specialized cells known as neurons.

NEURONS, SYNAPSES, NEUROTRANSMITTERS, AND NEURORECEPTORS

The neuron is the specialized cell that makes up the tissue of the nervous system. In the human brain there are around 80,000 million neurons interconnected through a huge tangle of physical "wires" that extend from their bodies and link them together to form a network. These wires, called axons (which are long and send messages) and dendrites (which are shorter and receive messages), allow communication between the cells through chemical and electrical signals.

These electrical impulses that travel through the neuron as if it were a wire are known as action potentials, and they could be compared to telegraph messages using Morse code. They are electrical impulses that can propagate within the neuronal "wiring" of the brain and travel long distances through the nerves of the body at very high speeds.

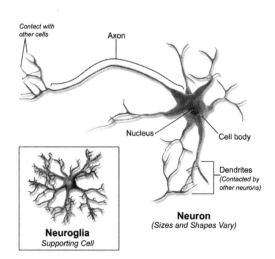

Morphological structure of a neuron. Image by Blausen. com staff, Medical gallery of Blausen Medical 2014, WikiJournal of Medicine.

In any cable network there must be "connectors" that link to each other and to other devices. In the nervous system, the connectors that link the axon of a sending neuron with the dendrites of a receiving neuron are known as synapses, and they are the points where neurons almost touch. But, as they do not really touch each other most of the time, upon reaching these points, the electricity that traveled through the axons (wires) makes some chemical signals "jump" from one neuron's axon to the next neuron's dendrite; these chemicals are the neurotransmitters. So, although neurons use electricity to send messages within the different parts of their elongated body, when it comes to passing that message to other neurons, they do so mostly by "splashing" each other with chemicals, called neurotransmitters, which are released when that message in the form of an electrical impulse reaches the end of the axon and must pass on to the next neuron. Although it seems impossible, this process that can seem so complex occurs in intervals of milliseconds, and each neuron can be connected to 10,000 others.

The chemical signals between neurons (neurotransmitters) are quite

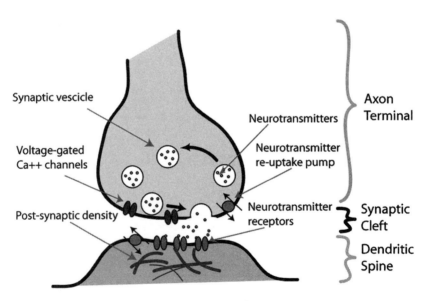

Simplified drawing of a synapse, where the axon of a neuron almost touches the dendrite of another neuron. Communication between the two is carried out by the release of chemical signals (neurotransmitters).
Image by Nrets. (See also color plate 1.)

varied and can send very different messages to the next neuron. We could say that they act as different "keys" that are released by the sending neuron (presynaptic neuron) to the synapse (the "connector") and will only fit in some specific "locks" (called neuronal receptors or neuroreceptors) of the receiving neuron (the postsynaptic neuron). Depending on the type of "doors" the sending neuron wants to open or close in the receiving neuron, the sending neuron will release one type of key or another.

The substances used by the body to send "non-nerve" messages over long distances or throughout the body are known as hormones,[2] while neurotransmitters are substances that also send messages but only between neurons and over very short distances in synapses, producing effects that can be immediate, short, and very localized, or propagated throughout the entire neural network. Some hormones that are generally used by the body can also be neurotransmitters, and some neurotransmitters behave like hormones. However, the key is that the electricity we generally associate with neurons and the nervous system in reality only occurs within each neuron; the communication between different neurons is fundamentally chemical and based on neurotransmitters, and they are involved in various processes. For example, some of the most famous neurotransmitters are serotonin, known to many as the "hormone of happiness" (although this is only partially true), or dopamine.

Just as there are multiple neurotransmitters that perform different functions, there are several types of neuroreceptors in the membranes of neurons, which are protein structures that act as locks for these "keys," and that are activated or not depending on the specific neurotransmitter (key) that comes close to them. For the same neurotransmitter there can be several subtypes of neuroreceptor, so it can even be said that some of them are "master keys" insofar as, sometimes, they not only can open a single lock but several of the same type, although they do not always turn equally well in all locks. In neuronal communication, what is ultimately important is not so much the neurotransmitter but what happens at the level of the receptors in the postsynaptic neuron, the locks that are being open, and how they do it.

---

2. For example, testosterone, adrenaline, insulin, cortisol, or melatonin.

These neurotransmitters and neuroreceptors can serve many different functions both inside and outside the brain, and, depending on the specific region of the brain or neuronal circuit on which they act, they can even be involved in completely opposite processes; so the generalization that a neurotransmitter only has a specific effect is overly simplistic and not always accurate. To give an idea of their diversity and the multiple processes in which they are involved, here are some neurotransmitters with their neuroreceptors and some of their main brain functions:

Neurotransmitter	Involved in processes of:	Neuroreceptors it acts upon:
Serotonin (5-HT)	Mood, sleep, hunger, anxiety, emotions, social behavior	5-HT1A, 5-HT1B, 5-HT1D, 5-HT1E, 5-HT1F, 5-HT2A, 5-HT2B, 5-HT2C, 5-HT4, 5-HT5A, 5-HT5B, 5-HT6, 5-HT7
Dopamine	Motivation, concentration, reward, pleasure, humor, euphoria	D1, D2, D3, D4, D5
GABA	Inhibition, relaxation, sleep	GABA-A, GABA-B
Norepinephrine (or epinephrine)	Related to action, concentration, fight-or-flight response	alpha-1, alpha-2, beta-1, beta-2, beta-3
Glutamate	Related to activation, learning, pain, memory, neuroplasticity	NMDA, Kainate, AMPA, mGluR1, mGluR5, mGluR2, mGluR3, mGluR4, mGluR6, mGluR7, mGluR8
Acetylcholine	Related to memory, motor skills, attention	Nicotinics (Nm, Nn), Muscarinics (M1, M2, M3)

Molecular Structure

Serotonin (5-HT).

Dopamine.

GABA.

Norepinephrine (or epinephrine).

Glutamate.

Acetylcholine.

There are many other neurotransmitters and neuroreceptors, as well as other types of molecules that can act as neurotransmitters, although they are not released in the same way, such as oxytocin (related to emotional bonding, childbirth, and breastfeeding) or endorphins (related to analgesia and acting on opioid receptors).

As we can see, all this is not as simple as saying that serotonin is the hormone of happiness, but rather that it acts as a modulator with various functions depending on which of its fourteen different receptors it is activating and in which brain region, or neural network, it is found. Other neurotransmitters with fewer receptors can fulfill functions that are easier to explain, such as glutamate, which activates neurons and increases their electrical excitability, or GABA, which "turns them off" or reduces their electrical excitability. But these effects at the neuronal level do not always translate to the entire brain, and the result also depends on the specific networks that are being activated or deactivated.

Why is it so important to talk about how neurons communicate in this book's introduction? Because it is this chemical communication between neurons that allows the brain and the other parts of the nervous system to carry out all their functions. Just as it happens inside a computer, the operation of which depends not only on the work of one

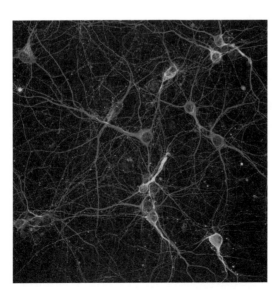

Network of neurons seen under the microscope. Image by ALol88. (See also color plate 2.)

of its parts but on the interaction (communication) between many of them, a neuron in our brain does not "think"; the neuronal network does. It is at this point that we can start talking about how exogenous molecules,[3] like psychoactive substances, influence these processes.

NEUROPHARMACOLOGY

A drug is a molecule that is considered "bioactive" because, due to its structure and chemical configuration, it can interact with protein macromolecules, generally called receptors (locks), located in the membrane, cytoplasm, or nucleus of a cell (such as neurons, for example), giving rise to an action and a noticeable effect. For example, when we take ibuprofen, it reduces pain and inflammation. For this reason, pharmacology is the branch of science that studies how the drug (be it a medicine bought in a pharmacy, a medicinal plant, or a beer served at a bar) interacts with the body—its actions, effects and properties.

Neuropharmacology in particular studies how some drugs act specifically on neurons and the nervous system. Drugs with the ability to interact with our neurons and nervous tissues are called "psychoactive substances" or "psychoactive drugs," and sometimes simply "drugs," and they cover a wide range of molecules such as alcohol, anxiolytics, analgesics, tobacco, cocaine, coffee, LSD, and MDMA.

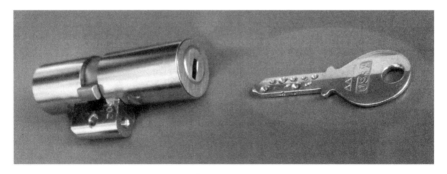

A lock and its key—an analogy of the interaction between drug–receptor or
neurotransmitter–neuroreceptor. Photo by ItalianLocksmith.

---

3. Produced outside the body.

Based on this definition we can begin to understand why the concept of neurotransmitter (key) and neuroreceptor (lock) is so important to understand, since psychoactive substances (both legal and illegal) act precisely there, on those locks in our neurons. They affect the interaction between our internal keys and locks, sometimes acting as if they were the keys themselves and opening those locks (agonistic effect), like how a pick or false key opens a lock in the absence of the original key. At other times they block them, as if they were broken keys that fit but do not turn, and not letting other keys in (antagonistic effect). Also, sometimes, they simply make the neurons unable to withdraw those keys after releasing them (reuptake inhibitors), or even "release" more keys than expected (transporter reversals). All these possible actions of drugs in the synapse are what give us such a wide range of possible effects, causing neuronal activations or preventing them, in a way that is different from the normal functioning of the system. They are said to have a certain affinity (or fit) for one or more neuroreceptors at a time and can bind to them with lesser or even greater affinity (strength) than our own neurotransmitters.

In essence, it could be said that psychoactive substances act as if they were our own neurotransmitters, but instead of being generated within our own body (endogenous), they enter our body from the outside (exogenous), and their way of interacting with neuroreceptors is different from that of our own neurotransmitters.

This happens at the neuronal level, but if we see what happens at the brain level, these changes in the locks of our neurons have a global impact that temporarily changes the way the brain works and may affect the way different brain regions communicate with each other, over-activating some regions, turning off others, or causing incoordination in others (see, for example, color plate 3). This is what produces the changes in consciousness that we notice, for example, when we drink a beer, drink coffee, or consume any other substance with psychoactive properties.

Although much remains to be discovered about the neurochemical processes that form the basis of our consciousness, every day we know more about the basic neurochemistry of our brain functions, the organ that lays the biological foundations of our thoughts, feelings, and behaviors. Therefore, every day we have a better understanding of how drugs influence them, and how we can use them to advance science and therapies.

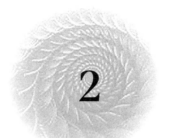

Introduction to Psychoactive Substances

TALKING ABOUT PSYCHOACTIVE SUBSTANCES

In the previous chapter, we saw that psychoactive substances (also known as psychoactive drugs) are those that, upon entering the body (via any route: oral, nasal, intramuscular, intravenous), exert a direct effect on the central nervous system, causing specific changes to its functions (perceptions, thoughts, emotions, behavior, pain, state of mood, etc.). Examples of these substances include alcohol, caffeine, anxiolytics, antidepressants, painkillers, and other psychoactive drugs, including some of the illicit kind.

When we speak of illicit psychoactive drugs we are referring, of course, to those whose production, trafficking, or sale has been illegalized. If we were to ask about them on the street, the first thing people would comment on would be their addictive, harmful, and, in certain circumstances, even deadly nature. Yet, these characteristics are not intrinsic to these substances, but rather depend largely on the use that is made of them.

So, when talking about psychoactive substances or psychoactive drugs, if they are not all illegal, not all addictive, not all harmful, what do they have in common? What identifies them as a family and differentiates them from all other drugs or any other known substance?

As we began to see in the previous chapter, it all comes down to where they act and what effects they produce.

What all the molecules mentioned above have in common is their ability to directly influence neuronal activity in the central nervous system. Psychoactive substances act on the neuroreceptors of these neurons (or on the neurotransmitters that allow them to communicate with each other), resulting in psychoactive effects of various kinds, like modifying our consciousness, mood, and level of alertness. Drugs, whether legal, restricted for medical use, or illegalized,[1] are those keys that, like our internal neurotransmitters, fit into the locks of our neurons (or act on our internal keys).

Therefore, if we want to be more precise when referring to substances such as alcohol, cannabis (marijuana), cocaine, or LSD ("acid"), ideally, we should not just talk about drugs, which is a very broad term, but "psychoactive substances" or "psychoactive drugs." These terms are essentially synonyms. In addition to being synonyms, they are the most precise terms to use. However, to make it easier for the reader and keeping with the usual social lexicon, throughout this book we will use the word "drug" (and "substance") as an abbreviated form of "psychoactive drug" or "psychoactive substance."

Far from technical definitions, drugs, whether legal, illegalized, or restricted for medical use, are fundamentally known for their effects on the mind and behavior. They are tools that not only stimulate or relax us, but also they allow us to access other altered or non-ordinary states of consciousness.

The science that studies the effects of these substances on the mind—cognition, emotions, thoughts, perceptions, motivations, and behaviors—is known as "psychopharmacology."

---

1. Instead of talking about legal and illegal drugs, the author prefers to discuss legal drugs, drugs restricted for medical use, or "illegalized" drugs. This distinction between illegal and illegalized is made because the legal status of a drug is not an intrinsic characteristic but, rather, it derives from a social construction, such as laws, which are subject to constant change. Drugs, like any other natural element, are "legal" in principle until society, through its governments and legislators, decides otherwise. Drugs were not created illegal, nor did they exist being illegal and then legalized—quite the opposite; they existed and were legal (in the natural world or when they were created by the hand of man) and later, rulers and legislators decided to restrict some of them for medical use and others were directly illegalized for most uses except very controlled research.

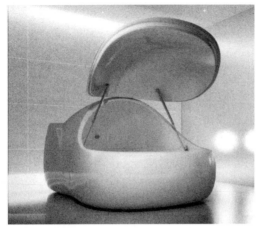

Sensory isolation tank, where you float in body-temperature salt water in the dark, in silence to deprive the brain of any sensory input and achieve an altered state of consciousness. Photo by Floatguru.

Fortunately, psychoactive substances are not the only tool we have to access these altered states of consciousness. There are various ancient and modern practices that allow us to achieve states that can resemble those obtained through psychoactive substances, such as meditation, breathing, fasting, extreme sports, sleep deprivation, sensory isolation chambers,[2] or lucid dreaming.[3] People who enjoy exploring altered states of consciousness through these various pharmacological or non-pharmacological tools are known as "psychonauts" and the discipline they practice as "psychonautics."

TYPES OF PSYCHOACTIVE SUBSTANCES

What do a boat, a car, a plane, and a bicycle have in common? Not all of them have wheels, or motors, or move on the same surface, or at the same speed, or work the same. However, we can say that, in essence, they are all vehicles whose function is to move people, other living beings, or things. However, if we wanted to go beyond a generic description, we would be making a mistake by referring to all vehicles in the same terms, without

---

2. Sensory isolation chambers or tanks seek to minimize the information provided by the senses to the brain through a combination of darkness, silence, absence of odors, and bodily comfort. They were very popular in the 1960s and 1970s thanks to the work of neuropsychiatrist John C. Lilly and the movie *Altered States*.
3. Lucid dreams are those in which the person is aware of dreaming and takes control.

distinguishing their different functions and characteristics and without considering the different security measures that we must employ prior to using them.

The same goes for drugs. When we hear about them as a whole, one of the first things we should keep in mind is that we are talking about a group of very heterogeneous chemical substances and, although they each act on the nervous system and can alter our perception, emotions, mental processes, and behavior, they act in different ways, intensities, and directions, and they carry different risks.

Moreover, as it is not possible (nor functional) to carefully test or study each drug and their effects one by one in order to talk about them, we inevitably need "classification models" to arrange what they have in common and what differentiates them—a way of systematically grouping psychoactive substances that allows us to know their main effects and risks, and thus be able to speak, properly this time, of types of drugs.

Currently, it is very common for the general population to be guided by the classification system dictated by the legal status of substances, something that is not very informative, is susceptible to change, and has no scientific basis. This approach to drugs basically tells us that substances are divided into a small group of "legal drugs," such as alcohol, coffee, and tobacco (which many people do not even consider drugs), and another enormous group of "illegal drugs"[4] (or simply "drugs" for most), such as cocaine and MDMA. If we were to ask on the street about how we can somehow classify illegal drugs, many people would apply a subdivision based on their own subjective perception of the risk they pose, dividing them into "soft drugs" and "hard drugs," which is another arbitrary classification based on press headlines, rumors, or the more or less well-founded opinion of each individual.

Also, you may be surprised to discover that many of the "drugs" you probably think are hard or totally illegal today turn out to have authorized medical use. In fact, drugs with such gloomy and stigmatized names as "liquid ecstasy" (GHB), "speed" (amphetamine), "heroin" (diamorphine), "crystal meth" (methamphetamine), fentanyl,

---

4. People don't usually say "illegalized drugs."

and ketamine are authorized for medical use and currently marketed under names such as Xyrem, Adderall, Desoxyn, Actiq, Duragesic, and Ketalar, and they are dispensed in pharmacies or hospitals on a daily basis, just as cocaine, opium, LSD and many others once were.

Probably, some people would also allude to the usual classification between natural or synthetic drugs that, contrary to popular belief, tells us very little about their effects and their risks. In fact, many substances that were believed to be only synthetic are not, such as GHB ("liquid ecstasy"), which later turned out to be naturally occurring not only in wine, vermouth, or berries, but also in our brains and the brains of other mammals.

On the other hand, if we go to a more academic field, we can find more technical answers generally related to the different chemical structures of substances, such as tryptamines, phenylethylamines, or cathinones, which are tremendously complex classifications to handle for practical or informative purposes.

Luckily, for those people who are really interested in learning the main intrinsic characteristics of psychoactive substances, in a rigorous yet simplified and useful way, classifications based on their effects have existed since ancient times, the richness and complexity of which are advancing through science and experimentation.

Until the end of the last century, the classification based on their main effects was very simple, and it was limited to dividing drugs into stimulants, sedatives, and hallucinogens, which could be represented graphically in a triangle, square, or star depending on whether some combined categories were added, such as stimulant–psychedelic or depressant–psychedelic drugs. Derek Snider created an excellent graphical depiction of these relationships with four overlapping spheres (see color plate 4), and the infographic by David McCandless "Drugs World"[5] allows us to clearly see the different profiles of effects that sometimes occur in the same molecule. The image prepared by the NGO Espolea (Mexico), baptized as *El Universo de las Drogas*[6] [the universe of drugs], depicts a four-pointed star.

---

5. David McCandless, "Drugs World" (September 2010), via the Information is Beautiful website.
6. "What is the Universe of Drugs?" (January 2016), via the International Consortium of Drug Policy website.

As some parts of these graphs were confusing, over time basic categories were added and subdivided (for example, the group of sedatives became divided into depressants and analgesics). However, starting in 2010, the limitations of such a rudimentary classification began to be seen very clearly with the explosion of the market of "research chemicals," new illegal synthetic drugs inspired by already banned molecules, some even described as far back as the 1980s in books such as the *PiHKAL*[7] and the *TiHKAL*,[8] and that were sold freely on the internet and in "smartshops" during the time it took them to be illegalized. Many of these substances were assigned to the "miscellaneous" or "other" category, or were placed in mixed sections, as has always been the case with MDMA or ecstasy (the effects of which were located at the intersection of stimulants and psychedelics), or cannabis, which used to be placed between depressant and psychedelic.

In 2012 in the United Kingdom, a new classification model was developed by Mark Adley, U.K. Drugwatch, and several members in psychonaut forums who managed to solve, to a great extent, the limitations of the old systems through the creation of three new categories: empathogenic/entactogenic, cannabinoids, and dissociative, updating the term hallucinogens to psychedelics, and the term analgesics to opioids. They decided to place all seven categories of substances in a circle, and "The Drugs Wheel" was born[9] (see color plate 6)—probably the best effects-based drug classification model that we have today for basic drug knowledge, and one that combines simplicity with rigor by classifying most of the established drugs and many of the new synthetic substances (or new psychoactive substances, NPS)[10] in these seven categories of effects.

---

7. Alexander Theodore Shulgin and Ann Shulgin, *Pihkal: A Chemical Love Story* (Berkeley: Transform Press, 1991).

8. Alexander Theodore Shulgin and Ann Shulgin, *Tihkal: The Continuation* (Berkeley: Transform Press, 1997).

9. Available in multiple versions and translations on The Drugs Wheel website.

10. A new psychoactive substance (NPS) is a drug that has been recently made available and/or popularized and is designed to mimic the effects of established illegal drugs, yet it is not controlled by international drug conventions yet.

Based on this simple classification of drugs according to their effects, let's define each of the seven categories, their main uses, and their risks.

STIMULANTS

Stimulants are mainly those substances that activate, energize, cause euphoria, increase concentration, and raise alertness. In most cases they do this through their direct or indirect action on the neurotransmitters dopamine and norepinephrine, their neuroreceptors, or their systems. These substances tend to increase brain activation, which is why they are called "stimulants." Some examples of this category are:

- Caffeine (coffee, tea, energy drinks)
- Cocaine ("coke," "blow")
- Amphetamines ("speed," Adderall)
- Methamphetamines ("meth," Desoxyn)
- Nicotine (tobacco)
- MDPV ("cannibal drug")
- Alpha-PVP ("flakka")

Main Uses
Some stimulants such as methylphenidate or amphetamine are used in medicine to treat attention-deficit/hyperactivity disorder (ADHD) and

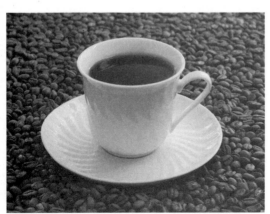

Caffeine from coffee or tea is the most famous and consumed stimulant in the world. Photo by Zacharias Korsalka.

narcolepsy[11] or to accompany treatments that can cause drowsiness (caffeine, pseudoephedrine, etc.). Stimulants were commonly used in the past to accelerate weight loss in specific cases (amphetamines and methamphetamines), or as bronchodilators (amphetamines) or local anesthetics (cocaine).

They are also used as nootropics, or cognitive enhancers, in academia and in the workplace. In fact, caffeine is the most used stimulant worldwide, with millions of doses consumed daily, followed by the next widely consumed stimulant, nicotine, in the form of tobacco.

They are also widely used alone or combined, at a recreational level, in leisure spaces such as nightclubs and festivals, as well as other illegalized stimulants such as cocaine or amphetamine.

Main Risks

All drugs have risks, stimulants included. This does not mean that most of these risks are always inherent to the substance itself but rather that an important derivation of the use that is made of them, influenced by important variables related to the substance itself (like type, dose, frequency, purity, adulterations, and route of administration), to the user (state of physical and mental health, psychological state, emotional state, intention, tolerance, combinations with other drugs) and the context of use (social context, legal status, risky activities, driving). Therefore, these risks will depend on many variables and, most of the time, can be reduced, although they can never be completely ruled out except by abstaining.

In the worst cases, the use of stimulants can lead to cardiovascular problems (such as heart attacks, arrhythmia, tachycardia, high blood pressure, strokes, or other cerebrovascular accidents), dehydration and hyperthermia ("heat stroke"), hyponatremia,[12] seizures, or transient psychological problems such as insomnia, anxiety, paranoia, and even stimulant psychosis.[13]

---

11. Disease that makes it difficult to regulate sleep-wake cycles, causing people to suffer from extreme sleepiness at any time of the day.
12. Condition where sodium levels are low due to excess water, lack of nutrition, and drug-altered urinary excretion; very rare but dangerous.
13. Stimulants at high doses can produce psychosis in predisposed people; an episode of transient psychosis called "stimulant psychosis" or "toxic psychosis" can result in poorly rested people.

Likewise, accidents can occur as a result of the euphoria and recklessness produced by the substance (which makes driving a dangerous activity), and in certain people and conditions, they can produce antisocial behavior such as aggression.

Some stimulants can cause hangovers, neurotoxicity, or emotional comedowns, especially in high doses or when mixed with alcohol or other drugs.

The long-term risks of stimulant use are highly dependent on the type of stimulant, the person using it, the frequency of use, and the doses taken. High frequency or high doses can lead to physical tolerance, psychological addiction, neuropsychiatric abnormalities, and cardiovascular diseases such as cardiomyopathy. The use of some types of stimulants can be highly addictive, both physically and psychologically, and faster routes of administration (such as injection, vaporization, or insufflation) are often more problematic than slower routes (oral administration). Neural adaptations to long-term effects can also be problematic, making it difficult to quit after chronic use.

DEPRESSANTS

Substances that mainly relax, disinhibit, sedate, slow down the mind, and cause euphoria are considered depressants, generally due to their action on GABA neuroreceptors. They reduce neuronal and cerebral activation; hence their designation as "depressants." Paradoxically, depressant substances, at low doses, tend to produce a feeling of energy and euphoria, which is actually because the first brain regions to slow down their activity are the most evolved ones, like the prefrontal cortex, in charge of inhibitions and social norms, leading to disinhibition and losing control over more primitive regions of the brain and their associated behaviors. Some examples are:

- Alcohol (beer, wine, rum, gin, whiskey, vodka, other liquors)
- Benzodiazepines (alprazolam, lorazepam, diazepam, Orfidal, Valium, Trankimazin)
- Barbiturates

- GHB (or its precursor, GBL) misnamed "liquid ecstasy" (and "G," "juice," Xyrem)
- 2M2B
- Mebroqualone

Main Uses

Depressant drugs are used in medicine as anxiolytics, muscle relaxants, sedatives, hypnotics, and anesthetics.

Outside the medical world, they are widely used in the recreational field for their disinhibiting and social properties, with alcohol being one of the three most consumed drugs in the world, behind coffee (caffeine) and tobacco (nicotine).

There have also been uses in the criminal field as a chemical submission[14] tool or "rape drugs."

Main Risks

As we commented with respect to stimulants, the risks of depressant drugs will depend a lot on the aforementioned variables of the substance itself, the user, and the context—risks that can be reduced but never completely eliminated, except by abstaining.

In the worst cases, the consumption of depressants can lead to dizziness, vomiting, coma, and even cardiorespiratory arrest.

Some depressants such as GHB/GBL or benzodiazepines (especially if they are not sold already in doses) have high pharmacological potency, so accidental overdoses can occur. They can also facilitate accidents due to their effects on coordination and reflexes (driving or any motor activity can be dangerous). Depressant substances, such as alcohol, can also cause aggression and recklessness in some people.

Some depressants can be toxic, especially in high doses, or if they are mixed with other substances. In the case of alcohol, it is common for it to produce a multifactorial phenomenon known as a "hangover" that is derived from a combination of lack of rest, dehydration, stomach

---

14. Chemical submission is to drug a victim to facilitate a crime such as robbery, sexual assault, or kidnapping.

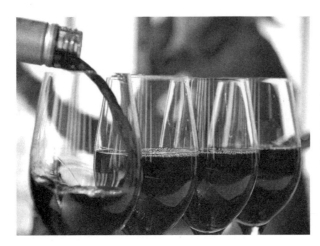

Red wine glasses. Alcohol is the most widely known and consumed depressant in the world. Photo by Maria Eklind.

irritation, toxic effects on the brain and liver, headache, neuroinflammation, nausea, and neuroadaptive effects.

The long-term risks of using depressant substances depend very much on the type, the person, the frequency of use, and the dose. High frequency or high doses can lead to addiction, liver and brain damage (particularly from alcohol), cardiovascular disease, cancer, and neurotoxicity.

Depressants can be physically and psychologically addictive. Furthermore, since some are widely available and accepted in many societies, such as alcohol or benzodiazepines, the social context may mask addiction or encourage increased consumption, especially in the case of alcohol.

If the consumption of depressants such as alcohol is maintained over time, the brain can develop adaptations that make it dangerous to stop abruptly. In the case of alcohol, a syndrome known as "delirium tremens" may develop, which could even lead to death. Because of this, slow and well-planned detoxification or the use of other depressant psychoactive drugs is often temporarily necessary to taper off. This chronic consumption also takes its toll on many areas of the brain, especially those related to memory, and can produce forms of dementia, such as the well-known Wernicke-Korsakoff syndrome, which is related to an alcohol-induced deficiency of thiamine (vitamin B1). Not only does the brain suffer from chronic alcohol consumption, but this condition is also particularly damaging to the liver. In cases of chronic consumption, fatty liver, cirrhosis, or liver failure may occur. Long-term alcohol consumption is also related to cardiovascular and metabolic diseases.

OPIOIDS

Opioids are those substances that produce sensations of analgesia (physical and emotional), well-being, or euphoria through their action on opioid receptors in the brain, emulating the effect of endorphins. Their name comes from its similarity to the substances present in opium, such as morphine. As with depressants, although their action is fundamentally inhibitory, at low doses they produce a subjective sensation of stimulation. Some examples are:

- Morphine (opium, poppy)
- Heroine ("dope," "smack," "junk")
- Codeine ("cody," "lean," "sizzurp," "purple drank")
- Methadone ("mud," "amidone," "methadose," and "done")
- Buprenorphine
- Tramadol ("trammies," "ultras")
- Fentanyl ("fent," "fenty," "apache")
- Ocfentanil
- MT-45

Main Uses
Some opioid drugs are used in medicine as analgesics, anesthetics, antitussives, or antidiarrheals.

Drug policy has always had a complicated relationship with opioids since they are very addictive substances but very necessary and difficult to substitute in the treatment of pain.

Main Risks
As we commented with respect to stimulants and depressants, the risks of opioid drugs will depend on the variables of the substance itself, the user, and the context—risks that can be reduced but never completely eliminated, except by abstaining.

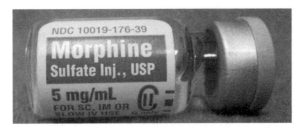

Bottle of morphine for hospital use, the best-known natural opioid.
Photo by Vaprotan.

In the worst cases, opioid use can lead to dizziness, vomiting, coma, or even cardiorespiratory arrest.

Most opioids are pharmacologically very potent and have a low safety ratio, so accidental overdoses can easily occur if their purity, adulteration, and dosage are unknown. Fortunately, this class of drugs has a specific antidote: naloxone.

In the long term, opioids are highly addictive substances that generate tolerance very quickly, so their therapeutic use should be as short as possible.

It is worth mentioning that some common routes of administration of opioids, such as intravenous injection, can present risks themselves in certain contexts, such as the transmission of diseases like hepatitis or HIV if sterile equipment is not used.

CANNABINOIDS

Cannabinoids are those substances that produce calm, time and sensory distortions, creativity, laughter, and other effects through their action on cannabinoid neuroreceptors in the brain and other areas of the body. Their name comes from the *Cannabis sativa* plant. Some examples of cannabinoids include the active ingredients of cannabis, THC (tetrahydrocannabinol) and CBD (cannabidiol), of which THC is the most responsible for cannabis's psychoactive effects while CBD has a modulating action; in the field of new psychoactive substances, we can also find a string of new synthetic cannabinoids, such as 5C-AKB48 and MDMB-4en-PINACA, and semisynthetic cannabinoids, like HHC (hexahydrocannabinol).

Main Uses

In recent decades, much research has been done on the therapeutic use of cannabis and cannabinoids for the treatment of different diseases, and there is a growing number of countries or regions that have already authorized their medical use for conditions such as chronic pain, Parkinson's, chemotherapy nausea, epilepsy, glaucoma, cancer, and PTSD. Its nonmedical use is also widespread, being considered the most widely used illegalized drug in the world.

Main Risks

As with previous substances, the risks of cannabinoid drugs will depend a lot on the variables of the substance itself, the user, and the context— risks that can be reduced but never completely eliminated, except by abstaining.

At the risk level, it is convenient to establish a clear distinction between natural cannabinoids present in *C. sativa* and those of synthetic origin, sometimes called "spice."

In the worst cases, the use of natural cannabinoids could lead to anxiety, paranoia, psychotic episodes, or other mental disorders in predisposed

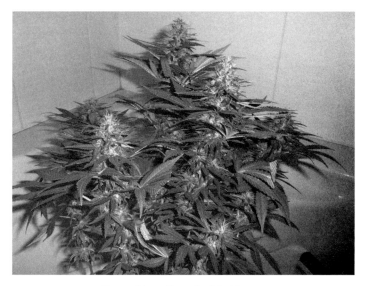

Cannabis sativa plant in bloom.
Photo by Pavel Sevela. (See also color plate 25.)

individuals. It can be difficult to know if someone is at risk of a psychotic reaction, especially if someone is still very young, which is one of the reasons why the use of cannabinoids is generally less risky in older and more mature people than in teenagers.

Although on a physical level it is generally considered safe, high doses can produce a "whitey" or "green out," characterized by paleness, nausea, cold sweat, tachycardia, hypotension, or dizziness, which are risks for people with heart problems. Nevertheless, it is not considered toxic at a physiological level, and, despite its large consumer base, deaths associated with cannabis are almost nonexistent except in very specific situations. One of the most common adverse effects is the above mentioned "green out," episodes of dizziness and transient discomfort normally associated with high doses. Still, as we have seen, they have psychological risks, being able to precipitate the manifestation of psychotic disorders in predisposed people.

A common risk in the consumption of cannabis is the overdose associated with consuming it orally in the form of edibles or cannabis cooking, with better absorption and potency being much greater by this route. In addition, since it takes several hours for the effects to be noticed when being ingested orally, there are cases of re-dosing due to impatience, which can produce an overdose that, although not fatal, can be a long and unpleasant experience.

Regarding synthetic cannabinoids, they are new, unknown, and extremely powerful substances, pharmacologically speaking, so it is very easy to accidentally overdose on them and expose yourself to risks much greater than those of natural cannabis consumption.

EMPATHOGENS/ENTACTOGENS

Empathogens, or entactogens, are substances that have the peculiarity of generating mostly empathy, love, and connection with other people and with oneself, as well as positive emotions, well-being, sociability, and emotionality by releasing large amounts of serotonin from our neurons, as well as dopamine, norepinephrine, oxytocin, and other neurotransmitters.

The word "empathogen" alludes to its ability to generate empathy, while "entactogen" is derived from the root *en* (Greek for "within"), *tactus* (Latin for "tactile") and *gen* (Greek for "produce"), that is, to produce contact with oneself, to connect with oneself. Both words refer to this specific class of drugs led by MDMA, but the former term (empathogen) was proposed initially by the psychologist Ralph Metzner to highlight the empathy component of the drugs' effect, while the latter term (entactogen) was proposed by biochemist David Nichols to expand the term beyond the drugs' empathetic effect, move away from the negative connotations of the root *páthos* (Greek for "suffering" or "passion"), and avoid any association with the term "pathogenesis" (meaning the origination and development of a disease).

These substances can also have stimulant and psychedelic properties at high doses but are not distinguished by them (this is why some empathogen/entactogen substances like MDMA are also considered to be semi-psychedelic or atypical psychedelics). The main substances in this category are:

- MDMA ("ecstasy," "molly," "XTC," "adam")
- MDA ("love pill," "sass," "sassafras")
- 6-APB ("benzofury")
- MDMC ("methylone," "explosion," "bk-MDMA")

Main Uses

Currently, empathogenic/entactogenic drugs do not have an officially authorized medical use, except in some cases in Australia. The United States might be the first country to formally authorize and commercialize MDMA for PTSD in the next few years through the FDA. Since MDMA is already in the final stages of clinical research, its compassionate use for certain cases can be requested in some countries already.

The recreational use of empathogens such as MDMA is widespread in leisure spaces such as music festivals, concerts, or nightclubs, but also for social, emotional, and sexual relationships.

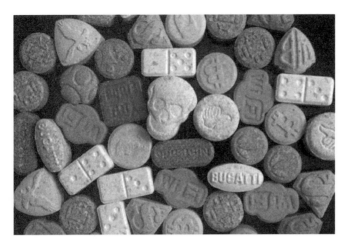

Ecstasy pills (MDMA), the most famous empathogenic/ entactogenic substance.

Main Risks

As with all other previous substances, the risks of empathogenic/entactogenic drugs will depend a lot on the variables of the substance itself, the user, and the context—risks that can be reduced but never completely eliminated, except by abstaining.

In the worst cases, the consumption of empathogens/entactogens can lead to cardiovascular risks (such as heart attacks, strokes, arrhythmia, tachycardia, high blood pressure), hyperthermia (heat stroke), dehydration, or hyponatremia (low sodium levels and excess of water), interactions with other substances or medications, and accidents derived from the euphoria produced by the substance.

In the specific case of empathogens/entactogens, given their relationship with the serotonin system, it is especially important to control body temperature and hydration to avoid a heat stroke. Likewise, avoid overdoing it with excessive water or non-isotonic drinks, since there is also a risk of hyponatremia.

If taking high doses, re-dosing, or combining it with other substances, MDMA can produce nausea and vomiting, and a hangover can occur after a day or two. This hangover is characterized by being very emotional and can manifest itself as sadness, tiredness, emptiness, restlessness, or melancholy that does not usually last more than a day but can last longer.

The long-term risks of MDMA use depend very much on the frequency and doses consumed. High frequency or high doses can facilitate the onset of psychological disorders such as depression, cardiovascular disease, and even addiction, because, although not to the same extent as other stimulants, long-term abuse of MDMA does present some risk of psychological and physical addiction. Also, some degree of neurotoxicity seems to be another problem associated with the chronic use of high doses, but its extent and clinical implications are still debated.

Although uncommon, MDMA could sometimes induce anxiety, confusion, and delirium, especially if used without adequate preparation and in uncontrolled settings. The risk of having a psychotic reaction is extremely low and has not been shown to be a risk for healthy people, so it could be greatly minimized by avoiding the use of empathogens/entactogens in people with known psychosis, bipolarity, psychotic disorders, or a family history of these mental issues. It can be difficult to know if someone is at risk of a psychotic reaction, especially if someone is still very young, which is one of the reasons why the use of substances with psychedelic-like effects is generally less risky in older and more mature people and in controlled clinical settings with appropriate professional supervision.

Despite popular belief, numerous population studies[15] with sample sizes in the hundreds of thousands of people have shown that at the population level there is no correlation between the use of MDMA or psychedelics and mental illness of any kind.[16] In fact, the correlation indicates that the use of MDMA or psychedelics is associated with better mental health, less stress,[17] less depression,[18] and fewer suicidal

15. Teri S. Krebs and Pål-Ørjan Johansen, "Psychedelics and Mental Health: A Population Study," *PLoS One* 8, no. 8 (August 2013): e63972.

16. Pål-Ørjan Johansen and Teri Suzanne Krebs, "Psychedelics not Linked to Mental Health Problems or Suicidal Behavior: A Population Study," *Journal of Psychopharmacology* 29, no. 3 (March 2015): 270–79.

17. Peter S. Hendricks et al., "Classic Psychedelic Use Is Associated with Reduced Psychological Distress and Suicidality in the United States Adult Population," *Journal of Psychopharmacology* 29, no. 3 (March 2015): 280–88.

18. Grant M. Jones and Matthew K. Nock, "Lifetime Use of MDMA/Ecstasy and Psilocybin Is Associated with Reduced Odds of Major Depressive Episodes," *Journal of Psychopharmacology* 36, no. 1 (January 2022): 57–65.

thoughts.[19] Although correlation does not imply causation, these studies show that the image of MDMA or psychedelics as substances that cause mental illness or that attract people with mental illness is distorted by the media and by prevention campaigns based on fear.

DISSOCIATIVES

They are substances that mainly dissociate or separate us from our bodies, bring feelings of floating, numbness, and incoordination, generally by blocking glutamate receptors, and can have psychedelic properties at high doses (this is why some dissociative substances like ketamine are also considered to be semipsychedelic or atypical psychedelics). Some examples of this category include:

- Ketamine ("Special K," "Kit Kat," "K")
- PCP (phencyclidine)
- N2O ("laughing gas")
- MXE (methoxetamine)
- 2-FDCK

Main Uses
Some dissociative drugs are used in medicine as analgesics and anesthetics—for example, ketamine or laughing gas. Recently, a purification of one of ketamine's enantiomers,[20] esketamine, has been patented by the pharmaceutical company Janssen (part of Johnson & Johnson) and approved for the treatment of major depression, becoming the first compound with psychedelic effects approved for

---

19. Grant M. Jones and Matthew K. Nock, "MDMA/Ecstasy Use and Psilocybin Use Are Associated with Lowered Odds of Psychological Distress and Suicidal Thoughts in a Sample of U.S. Adults," *Journal of Psychopharmacology* 36, no. 1 (January 2022): 46–56.
20. An enantiomer is one of two molecules that are mirror images of each other but cannot be superimposed, much like left and right hands. In the case of ketamine, the two enantiomers are esketamine and arketamine, and regular ketamine is a mixture of both.

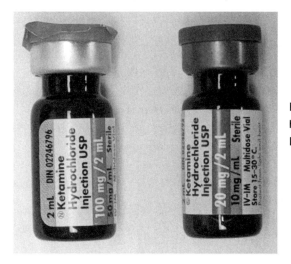

Bottles of ketamine for hospital use. Photo by Doc James.

the treatment of mental illness in the world, particularly in North America and Europe.

Its recreational use is also quite widespread; although originally associated with rave culture, in recent years its use has become popular in other leisure contexts and even the wellness industry.

Main Risks

As with all previous substances, the risks of dissociative drugs will depend a lot on the variables of the substance itself, the user, and the context—risks that can be reduced but never completely eliminated, except by abstaining.

In the worst cases, the use of dissociatives can lead to hypertension, dizziness, nausea, confusion, anxiety, fainting, and, since dissociative substances produce motor incoordination and loss of sensations, they are dangerous if there is a risk of falling or driving. At high doses they can produce an extreme dissociation experience known as "falling into a K-hole," which can be unpleasant. Very, very high doses of ketamine could cause death, but these doses are rare.

Like classic psychedelics, such as LSD or psilocybin, ketamine and nitrous oxide have low toxicity even at high doses. Therefore, physical and physiological safety is generally not a concern unless the person has accidentally taken a very high dose that could affect breathing, or if they drive, fall, faint, or engage in any other physically hazardous activity. Because ketamine slightly raises blood pressure and there is the possibility of intense experiences that can generate anxiety, people with a history of cardiovascular or psychiatric diseases should refrain from using it. Likewise, the continued use of nitrous oxide can lower the levels of vitamin B12 in the body and lead to neuronal problems, so it may pose a risk in people with low levels of this vitamin.

The main risk found in psychedelic experiences that can come from a high dose of ketamine is psychological, such as having a difficult experience ("bad trip"), a psychotic reaction that can occur in people with a predisposition or, in extremely rare cases, "flashbacks" (hallucinogen persisting perception disorder, or HPPD, although few cases are known). These risks increase at higher doses.

The probability of having a difficult experience or a bad trip is low and could be greatly minimized with a good set and setting. Long-lasting psychological difficulties resulting from such an experience (such as negative trauma, anxiety, or fear) are rare but can occur, especially if the substance is taken without prior experience in highly uncontrolled environments without adequate preparation of the user and their context (set and setting). Substances with psychedelic effects can amplify mental states, so using them with fear, worry, anxiety, or in uncomfortable or insecure contexts can make it easier to have bad experiences.

The risk of having a psychotic reaction is very low and has not been shown to be a risk for healthy people, so it could be greatly minimized by avoiding the use of ketamine in people with known psychosis, bipolar or psychotic disorders, or people with a family history of these mental disorders. It can be difficult to know if someone is at risk of a psychotic reaction, especially if someone is still young, which is one reason why the use of substances with psychedelic effects is generally less risky in older and more mature people and in controlled clinical settings with appropriate professional supervision.

Although the long-term risks of ketamine use depend very much on the frequency and the doses used, there are some specific long-term risks, such as addiction, tolerance, bladder damage, and urinary tract infections (common side effects of long-term ketamine abuse due to the way it is metabolized and excreted from the body), neurotoxicity, and withdrawal syndrome. But using them without considering underlying mental conditions such as psychosis, bipolarity, or psychotic disorders could worsen the course of these disorders and contribute negatively to the long-term outcome.

The neurotoxicity of ketamine is still debated, but it appears that it could produce some indirect excitotoxicity at very high doses and frequencies of use. However, it appears that no long-term cognitive impairments have been found to result from this, and short-term cognitive impairments appear to recover upon discontinuation of ketamine.

PSYCHEDELICS

"Classic" psychedelics, also called hallucinogens or entheogens, are substances that alter our perception and thinking, induce visions, amplify our senses, expand our consciousness, induce laughter, and increase our connection with nature and our inner self mainly by activating serotonin 5-HT2A neuroreceptors, although it is not always its main mechanism. Some psychedelic substances may also have stimulant or dissociative properties.

The term "psychedelic" derives from the Latin roots *psyche* (mind) and *delos* (to manifest); therefore the term refers to its ability to "manifest the mind" or the underlying mental processes, making them conscious.

Although the current official name is "psychedelic compound," "psychedelic drug," or "psychedelic substance," these substances have been given different names throughout history, such as hallucinogens, entheogens,[21] psychotomimetics, and there is currently a (longstanding) debate[22] about what the most appropriate terminology is, or whether to recover the term hallucinogenic. Since this work is primarily informative

---

21. C. A. Ruck et al., "Entheogens," *Journal of Psychedelic Drugs* 11, no. 1–2 (1979): 145–46.
22. Jonathan Ott, *Pharmacotheon: Entheogenic Drugs, Their Plant Sources and History* (United States: Natural Products Company, 1993).

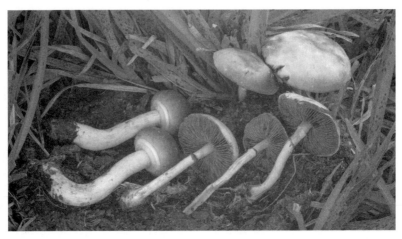

Psilocybe cubensis mushrooms, known as "magic mushrooms," a classic psychedelic. Photo by Alan Rockefeller.

in nature, we will stick primarily to current official terminology to avoid confusion, but these terms may be used interchangeably. Some examples of substances in this category are:

- LSD ("acid," "blotter," "dots," "microdots")
- Psilocybin (hallucinogenic mushrooms, magic mushrooms)
- Mescaline (peyote, San Pedro cactus)
- DMT ("Dimitri," changa, ayahuasca)
- 5-MeO-DMT ("toad")
- 1P-LSD
- 25i-NBOMe

Main Uses
Currently, in legislation, psychedelic substances are mostly considered high risk and have no authorized medical use, although this status is changing and we will talk about this extensively in this book.

Main Risks
As with previous categories, the risks of psychedelic drugs will depend a lot on the variables of the substance itself, the user, and the context—risks that can be reduced but never completely eliminated, except by abstaining.

When talking about risks, we can distinguish between those from psychedelic substances with a stimulant profile (such as DOC, DOM, DOI, 25i-NBOMe), which combine psychedelic and stimulant risks with "pure" psychedelics or "classics" like LSD, psilocybin, and DMT, which we will delve into in this book.

Classic psychedelics like LSD or psilocybin are substances with very low toxicity even at high doses, and in most cases no overdose deaths have yet been recorded in medical literature. Therefore, physical and physiological safety is generally not a concern beyond possible nausea or vomiting, unless the person is driving, falls, or engages in some other physically dangerous activity. In any case, and due to the possibility of intense experiences that can generate anxiety, people with a history of cardiovascular disease should refrain from using them.

The main risk found in psychedelic experiences is psychological, such as having a difficult experience or bad trip—a psychotic reaction that can occur in people with a predisposition—or in extremely rare cases, flashbacks (hallucinogen persisting perception disorder or HPPD, although few cases are known). These risks increase at high doses.

The probability of having a bad trip is low and could be greatly minimized with proper set and setting, as we will see later. Long-lasting psychological difficulties resulting from such an experience (such as negative trauma, long-lasting anxiety, or fear) are rare but can occur, especially if the substance is taken without prior experience in highly uncontrolled environments without adequate preparation of the user and their context (set and setting). Substances with psychedelic effects can amplify mental states, so using them with fear, worry, anxiety, or in uncomfortable or insecure contexts can make it more likely to have bad experiences.

The risk of having a psychotic reaction is very low and has not been shown to be a risk for healthy people, but rather for those with a propensity, so it could be greatly minimized by avoiding the use of psychedelics in people with known psychosis, bipolarity, or psychotic disorders, or people with a family history of these mental issues. It can be difficult to know if someone is at risk of a psychotic reaction, especially if someone is still very young, which is one reasons why the use of substances with psychedelic effects is generally less risky in older and more mature people and in controlled clinical settings with appropriate professional supervision.

Although the long-term risks of psychedelic use depend largely on the frequency, doses, and type of use, no specific long-term risks of psychedelic use are known due to their low potential for toxicity, low addictive potential, and high tolerance that prevents the creation of a habit (the desire to consume them usually decreases with use), and there is no withdrawal syndrome. Studies have found no detrimental effects in healthy people with long-term psychedelic use. But taking them despite underlying mental conditions such as psychosis, bipolar, or psychotic disorders is very risky and could worsen the course of these disorders and contribute negatively to long-term outcomes.

People who use psychedelics long-term tend to use them spaced across time and not regularly, as the experiences are very intense and require time to integrate and reflect upon. Tolerance also prevents frequent use, with potency reduced to half if consumed in the following days. It takes approximately three days of abstinence for tolerance to decrease by fifty percent and seven days to return to baseline in the absence of further consumption.

Despite popular belief, numerous population studies[23] with sample sizes in the hundreds of thousands of people have shown that, at the population level, there is no correlation between the use of MDMA or psychedelics and mental illness of any kind.[24] In fact, the correlation indicates that the use of MDMA or psychedelics is associated with better mental health, less stress,[25] less depression,[26] and fewer suicidal

---

23. Teri S. Krebs and Pål-Ørjan Johansen, "Psychedelics and Mental Health: A Population Study," *PLoS One* 8, no. 8 (August 2013): e63972.

24. Pål-Ørjan Johansen and Teri Suzanne Krebs, "Psychedelics not Linked to Mental Health Problems or Suicidal Behavior: A Population Study," *Journal of Psychopharmacology* 29, no. 3 (March 2015): 270–79.

25. Peter S. Hendricks et al., "Classic Psychedelic Use Is Associated with Reduced Psychological Distress and Suicidality in the United States Adult Population," *Journal of Psychopharmacology* 29, no. 3 (March 2015): 280–88.

26. Grant M. Jones and Matthew K. Nock, "Lifetime Use of MDMA/Ecstasy and Psilocybin Is Associated with Reduced Odds of Major Depressive Episodes," *Journal of Psychopharmacology* 36, no. 1 (January 2022): 57–65.

thoughts.[27] Although correlation does not imply causation, these studies show that the image of MDMA or psychedelics as substances that cause mental illness or attract people with mental illness is distorted by the media and by prevention campaigns based on fear, especially because these correlations do not occur, even taking into account that in the United States around thirty million people have tried psychedelics[28] and almost 6 million people took psychedelics in the United States in 2019.[29] The risks of these substances, although real, have been greatly exaggerated and very rarely produce lasting negative effects.[30] (See color plate 7 for a graphic summary of the drugs wheel with the effects and some risks of each of the drug categories mentioned in this chapter.)

27. Grant M. Jones and Matthew K. Nock, "MDMA/Ecstasy Use and Psilocybin Use Are Associated with Lowered Odds of Psychological Distress and Suicidal Thoughts in a Sample of U.S. Adults," *Journal of Psychopharmacology*, 36, no. 1 (January 2022): 46–56.

28. Teri S. Krebs and Pål-Ørjan Johansen, "Over 30 Million Psychedelic Users in the United States," *F1000Research* 2 (March 2013): 98.

29. Ofir Livne, Dvora Shmulewitz, Claire Walsh, Deborah S. Hasin, "Adolescent and Adult Time Trends in US Hallucinogen Use, 2002–19: Any Use, and Use of Ecstasy, LSD and PCP," *Addiction* 117, no. 12 (December 2022): 3099–3109.

30. Anne K. Schlag et al., "Adverse Effects of Psychedelics: From Anecdotes and Misinformation to Systematic Science," *Journal of Psychopharmacology* 36, no. 3 (March 2022): 258–72.

3

A History of Psychedelics in the West

PRE-LSD

It is not the purpose of this book to delve into humanity's rich, millennia-long history with psychedelic substances. It is an exciting topic but too extensive for the format of this book, and it has already been covered masterfully by other specialized works.[1] Therefore, I will focus especially on the Western scientific perspective and on what happened during the twentieth century and in recent decades, which have come to be known as the "psychedelic renaissance."

Although psychedelic substances have been used for millennia[2] for various sociocultural, political, and religious reasons, Western societies abandoned its use centuries ago. Throughout history, these substances have been linked to important aspects of societies, whether medicinal, spiritual, religious, divinatory, or ritualistic. In many cases they were the sacred sacrament of a religion or a god. Except for some explorers and

---

1. For example, *Plants of the Gods: Origins of Hallucinogenic Use* by Richard Evans Schultes and Albert Hofmann (1979); *Pharmacotheon: Entheogenic Drugs, Their Plant Sources and History* by Jonathan Otto (1993); and *Historia General de las Drogas* [The General History of Drugs] by Antonio Escohotado (1999).
2. Melanie J. Miller et al., "Chemical Evidence for the Use of Multiple Psychotropic Plants in a 1,000-Year-Old Ritual Bundle from South America," *Proceedings of the National Academy of Sciences of the United States of America* 116, no. 23 (May 2019): 11207–12.

intellectuals in recent centuries, few Westerners had contact with or interest in psychedelic substances until the end of the nineteenth century and, especially, the middle of the twentieth century, when science began to be interested in these mysterious substances.

Mescaline, the active ingredient in the peyote (*Lophophora williamsii*) and San Pedro (*Echinopsis pachanoi*) cacti, which had been used for thousands of years by Native Americans, was the first psychedelic substance (but not the first psychoactive drug) to be isolated and to enter Western science. The German pharmacologist Arthur Heffter isolated the active ingredients of peyote in 1897 and tested its psychedelic effects on animals and on himself.

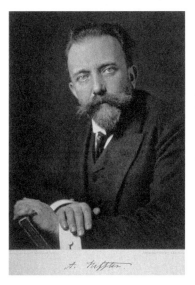

Arthur Heffter, who isolated the active principles of peyote in 1897, and whose psychedelic effects he also tested. Photo by Erwin Raupp, 1863–1931.

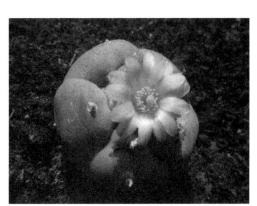

Peyote (*Lophophora williamsii*) one of the most famous mescaline containing cacti. Photo by MyName [Hans B.].

As early as 1919, the Austrian chemist Ernst Späth managed to synthesize mescaline. By then, some psychologists, such as the American Weir Mitchell, considered the father of neurology, and the Englishman Havelock Ellis, had already described their experiences with cacti. But it was the German American Heinrich Klüver who studied its effects in greater detail in the book *Mescal: And Mechanisms of Hallucinations*,[3] published in 1928, proposing its use to explore the unconscious.

POST-LSD

The event that marks the beginning of Western scientific interest in psychedelic substances happened on April 16, 1943, in Basel, Switzerland, where Dr. Albert Hofmann, researcher at Sandoz pharmaceutical laboratories, was working on synthetic derivatives of ergotamine (a compound present in the fungus *Claviceps purpurea,* known as ergot) in search of an analeptic (a stimulant for the respiratory and circulatory systems) when he began to feel unwell, to the point of needing to go home. As he wrote years later:

> . . . I was forced to interrupt my work in the laboratory in the middle of the afternoon and return home, being affected by a remarkable restlessness, combined with a slight dizziness. At home, I lay down and sank into a not unpleasant intoxicated-like condition, characterized by an extremely stimulated imagination. In a dreamlike state, with eyes closed (I found the daylight to be unpleasantly glaring), I perceived an uninterrupted stream of fantastic pictures, extraordinary shapes with intense, kaleidoscopic play of colors. After some two hours this condition faded away.[4]

The compound he was working on at the time was not entirely new, since it was a molecule that he himself had synthesized five years earlier:

---

3. Heinrich Klüver, *Mescal: And Mechanisms of Hallucinations* (University of Chicago Press, 1928).
4. Albert Hoffman, *LSD, My Problem Child* (New York: McGraw-Hill, 1980).

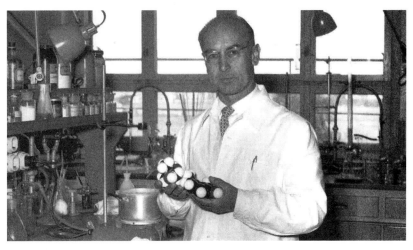

Albert Hofmann in his laboratory, holding a molecular model of his famous creation: LSD-25. Photo sourced via the Salte website (no longer accessible).

number twenty-five in a series of molecules derived from lysergic acid, lysergic acid diethylamide, annotated by its German acronym as LSD-25, but which had shown no interesting pharmacological properties in animal tests done in 1938 and had been discarded.

Intrigued by the origin of these strange effects that he had felt, and in case they could be due to some kind of accidental ingestion of that compound with which he was working, three days later, on April 19, he decided to do a little experiment on himself. He ingested a quarter of a milligram (or 250 millionths of a gram) of the compound, an amount that, at that time, was considered minuscule for any known compound and therefore of little risk, but that would prove to be a high dose in the case of this powerful new molecule.

Within half an hour, he began to feel strange again; his senses and his perception of things began to change. He felt like laughing and it was difficult for him to speak, so he asked his assistant Susi Ramstein to accompany him home. They rode their bicycles since it was his usual means of transport at the time, due to the restrictions on motor vehicles during World War II. Along the way, his condition intensified with strong visual and time distortions, so when he got home, fearing that he had been poisoned and that he was in danger, he asked that they bring him milk as a nonspecific antidote and that they call the doctor. After examining him, the doctor did not see that any of his vital signs were altered, and did not notice anything unusual in his condition, except for his two enormous pupils.

Seeing that his body was fine, that everything came from his mind, and that he would not die or be harmed, he began to feel calmer and more confident that he was not going insane.

Years later he described:

> ... little by little I could begin to enjoy the unprecedented colors and plays of shapes that persisted behind my closed eyes. Kaleidoscopic, fantastic images surged in on me, alternating, variegated, opening and then closing themselves in circles and spirals, exploding in colored fountains, rearranging and hybridizing themselves in constant flux. It was particularly remarkable how every acoustic perception, such as the sound of a door handle or a passing automobile, became transformed into optical perceptions. Every sound generated a vividly changing image, with its own consistent form and color. . . . [5]

The next day, after the experience, he felt tired but very well, renewed:

> I woke up next morning feeling refreshed, with a clear head, though still somewhat tired physically. A sensation of well-being and renewed life flowed through me. Breakfast tasted delicious and gave me extraordinary pleasure. When I later walked out into the garden, in which the sun shone now after a spring rain, everything glistened and sparkled in a fresh light. The world was as if newly created. All my senses vibrated in a condition of highest sensitivity, which persisted for the entire day. [6]

And, indeed, in a way, a new world had been created, because that April 19, 1943, would go down in history as "Bicycle Day," the first

---

5. Hoffmann, *LSD*.
6. Hoffmann, *LSD*.

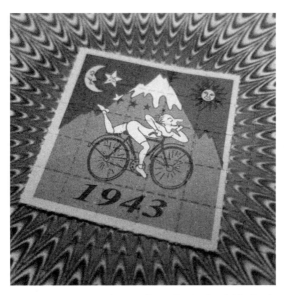

LSD blotter commemorating Bicycle Day: April 19, 1943. Each square of cardboard usually contains an impregnated dose of LSD that is between 100 and 150 micrograms, half of what Albert Hofmann took that day. Photo sourced via the Blotter Store website. (See also color plate 8.)

LSD trip in history, and the first psychedelic trip of a Western scientist in history that would become famous, ushering in a new era in neuroscience, psychotherapy, and spurring a sociocultural and political revolution that would ultimately lead to its own ban, as we'll see later.

After Albert Hofmann's discovery, the pharmaceutical company Sandoz began to thoroughly investigate this new and intriguing substance, patenting and marketing it under the name Delysid in 1947.

At a time when psychoanalytic paradigms prevailed in psychiatry, Sandoz began sending samples of LSD-25 to various universities, research centers, or individual therapists, offering to work with the substance, and asking them to send information about its possible applications. It soon began to be used to study schizophrenia because it was thought to be a psychotomimetic substance,[7] allowing psychiatrists to experience firsthand a state that was considered similar to psychosis, and to investigate brain neurochemistry, which in those years was very

---

7. Substance that emulates a psychosis.

poorly developed. The study of LSD sparked interest in other trypt-amines, a large family of compounds derived from the amino acid L-tryptophan, which includes endogenous neurotransmitters present in the human brain (such as serotonin or melatonin), and some psyche-delic compounds (such as psilocybin, psilocin, and dimethyltryptamine, or DMT) that, at the brain level, share their affinity for serotonin neu-roreceptors. In fact, the discovery of LSD had a great impact on the discovery and characterization of serotonin, in 1948, and on the study of the serotonergic system and its imbalances, in addition to fueling a change in the prevailing psychoanalytic paradigm on psychological and emotional disturbances toward a more neurochemical one.

Over the years, in the field of clinical psychiatry, a new use for LSD appeared in Europe: its therapeutic use in the form of psycholytic psy-chotherapy (meaning "mind loosening therapy"). It consisted in admin-istering successive low doses of LSD in psychoanalysis sessions, in order to facilitate patients' access to their experiences and progressively change their behavior patterns, but without the patient entering a deep psyche-delic experience. The term was coined by British psychiatrist Ronald A. Sandison, who had worked with LSD since 1952 and established the world's first dedicated LSD therapy unit at Powick Hospital in Worcestershire, England. In the development of psychotherapies with psychedelics in Europe, it is worth also mentioning the contribution of the Czech psychoanalyst Stanislav Grof, who would later develop transpersonal psychology, which works on altered states of conscious-ness using psychedelics or breathwork techniques.

In the early 1950s, at the Saskatchewan Hospital in Canada, the psychiatrist Humphry Osmond and the biochemist and psychiatrist Abram Hoffer formed a group dedicated to the biochemical investiga-tion of schizophrenia. This was a revolutionary idea at the time, com-pared to the prevailing conventional psychiatric practices, which gave it an exclusively psychological explanation. Humphry Osmond had already used mescaline as a psychotomimetic in the study of schizophre-nia, hypothesizing that schizophrenia could be caused by an autointoxi-cation with endogenous psychedelic products. In an attempt to improve his model of psychosis, he stockpiled every known psychedelic substance

LSD   **Serotonin**

Molecular structure of LSD compared to that of serotonin. Image from David E. Nichols, "Dark Classics in Chemical Neuroscience: Lysergic Acid Diethylamide (LSD)," *ACS Chemical Neuroscience* 9, no. 10 (October 17, 2018): 2331–43.

and continued self-experimentation until, finally, they decided to limit themselves to the use of LSD. They used LSD as a psychotomimetic on healthy individuals and thus tested treatments with them based on the premise that what worked with them while on LSD would also work with schizophrenia patients.

In 1954 in the same Saskatchewan Hospital, LSD also began to be used to treat thousands of alcoholic patients under the premise that it could help them in the beginning of their withdrawal process, by causing them experiences that could be similar to *delirium tremens*[8] to make them "hit rock bottom," to cause a dissuasive effect in a controlled way. This would help in their recovery process within the Alcoholics Anonymous program, avoiding the physical and social risks of reaching that same state with alcohol. But the results, far from producing this unpleasant effect, were that patients were enjoying the experience and even finding it revealing. The impact of the psychedelic experience was making it easier for alcoholics to identify their deep motivations for drinking, be able to work on them, and accept themselves as they were, and as a result, many were drinking less or quitting. Unbeknownst to them,

---

8. Alcohol withdrawal syndrome characterized by delusions, which can be fatal.

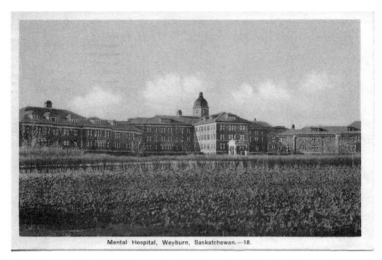

Mental Hospital, Weyburn, Saskatchewan.—18.

Saskatchewan Hospital. Courtesy of University of Saskatchewan, University Archives and Special Collections, Pamphlet Collection, LXX-1643, via The Canadian Encyclopedia website.

Abram Hoffer and Humphry Osmond were creating psychedelic-assisted psychotherapy, a new psychedelic-using psychotherapeutic approach that, unlike the prevailing psycholytic therapy in Europe, used large doses of LSD, in one or a few sessions, which invited introspection. The patient did not interact with the therapist during the psychedelic experience unless necessary, looking to reach "peak experiences" or "mystical experiences." At this point they had the collaboration of Alfred Hubbard, a self-proclaimed expert on psychedelics, who helped Osmond's team perfect their technique of working with psychedelic psychotherapy.

Within the three thousand patients who followed the treatment at the Saskatchewan Hospital, the rate of recovery obtained with severe alcoholics who achieved abstinence after one year of treatment reached fifty percent[9] compared to an effectiveness of twenty percent obtained in Alcoholics Anonymous in those years. Because of this, the cofounder of Alcoholics Anonymous, Bill Wilson, came to consider that the psychedelic experience could be a very valuable part in the process. Betty

---

9. J. Ross MacLean et al., "LSD-25 and Mescaline as Therapeutic Adjuvants," in *The Use of LSD in Psychotherapy and Alcoholism*, ed. Harold A. Abramson (Indianapolis: Bobbs-Merrill, 1967).

Eisner, a psychotherapist who worked with Bill Wilson, continued to perfect the model of the new psychedelic-assisted psychotherapy, together with her colleague Sidney Cohen by introducing the simultaneous work of two therapists (female and male) during the sessions where psychedelics were administered.

Something that almost all psychedelics have in common is the passion and interest that they have aroused in many people, to the point of creating "apostles" so fascinated with their therapeutic, spiritual, and scientific potential that they devoted themselves to the dissemination of their findings in different fields: scientific, political, therapeutic, and even social. Alfred Hubbard, also known as "Captain Hubbard," was one of the first great disseminators of LSD among the upper classes, politicians, and government officials, taking advantage of his enormous network of contacts. But then many more people with very similar goals would appear.

In 1952 Ernst Jünger published his book *Visit to Godenholm*,[10] in which he narrates his experiences with LSD, consumed with Albert Hoffmann a year before. But it did not receive much attention at the time. Quite the opposite of the famous English writer Aldous Huxley, to whom Humphry Osmond had supplied mescaline a year before, and who published *The Doors of Perception*[11] in 1954, a work that would begin to popularize psychedelics for the nonscientific public, a phenomenon of increasing popularization that would mark the following decades. The relationship between Huxley and Osmond would also bring about the term "psychedelic" in 1956. It was invented by Osmond by fusing the Greek words *psyche* (mind) and *deloun* (reveal, manifest); he later proposed it to Huxley in his letters. Despite the fact that the term "hallucinogenic" has always been widely used, the hallucinatory property as we currently understand it would only refer to one of the many possible characteristics of experiences with this type of substance, although there is still terminological debate on this.

---

10. Ernst Jünger, *Besuch Auf Godenholm* [Visit to Godenholm] (Germany, 1952).
11. Aldous Huxley, *The Doors of Perception and Heaven and Hell* (New York: Harper & Brothers, 1954 and 1956).

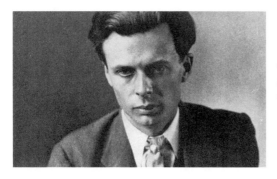

Aldous Huxley, author of *The Doors of Perception*, had a fascination with psychedelics.

Aldous Huxley, who was impressed with the potential of psychedelics and devoted much writing and public appearances to making them known, wrote:

> I suspect that these drugs [psychedelic drugs] are destined to play a role in human affairs at least as important as alcohol has hitherto, and incomparably more beneficial. . . . It enables one to know by experience that "God is love" feeling, that, in spite of death and suffering—everything is, in some way and in the final instance, all right.[12]

When he died of cancer in 1963, despite having been off psychedelics for several years, he asked to be given LSD on his deathbed, something that would soon begin to be tested on terminally ill patients, to help them lose their fear of death, accept their condition, reconcile with life, and enjoy their last months of existence.

In fact, the following year, a study by Erik Kast of the University of Chicago investigated the supposed analgesic power of LSD compared to common painkillers such as dihydromorphine and meperidine. In a group of fifty very sick patients with various pains mostly related to

---

12. The text comes from Aldous Huxley's essay "Drugs That Shape Men's Minds," originally published in the Saturday Evening Post in 1958. This essay was later included in the collection *Moksha: Aldous Huxley's Classic Writings on Psychedelics and the Visionary Experience* (Rochester VT: Park Street Press, 1999). In this essay, Huxley discusses the potential beneficial role of psychedelic drugs in society, comparing their potential positive impact to that of alcohol, but in a much more beneficial manner.

cancer, he observed an unexpected result by revealing that, in this type of patient, LSD produced a greater effect than those analgesics.[13] This result was highly surprising and would be almost implausible were it not for the researchers' observation that some of this analgesic power was not strictly pharmacological or physical, but rather seemed to come from an improvement in the patients' mood and from the reappraisal that some of them made of their terminal situation and the acceptance of their probable death.

This same author continued to carry out studies related to LSD and pain, but increasingly focused on other psychological parameters of his patients, such as their mood, their attitude towards their terminal state, their sleep patterns, their perception of pain, and noting that, with a single administration of LSD, positive changes were produced in these parameters that lasted more than three weeks. In successive studies, he continued to change his approach to study the influence that these experiences had on his patients in the religious and philosophical realm. To do this, he subjected terminally ill patients to the administration of a moderate dose of LSD, perceiving the changes mentioned in his previous studies. But what was peculiar in this case was that he also observed improvements in patient communication, along with feelings of unity and calm that lasted up to twelve days. With these studies, a new approach had just been born[14] that would have much future development: psychedelic-assisted psychotherapy for post-diagnostic terminal depression and its associated anxiety.

Based on these studies, and on the anecdotal observations of alcoholics who claimed to live an experience akin to death and resurrection under the effects of LSD, the psychiatrist Sidney Cohen expressed in an article in 1965 his intention to initiate a program of study of the palliative use of LSD as antidepressant therapy for terminal cancer patients, to allow them to lose their fear of the experience of death and improve

---

13. E. C. Kast and V. J. Collins, "Study of Lysergic Acid Diethylamide as an Analgesic Agent," *Anesthesia and Analgesia* 43 (May 1964): 285–91.
14. E. Kast, "LSD and the Dying Patient," *The Chicago Medical School Quarterly* 26, no. 2 (Summer 1966): 80–87.

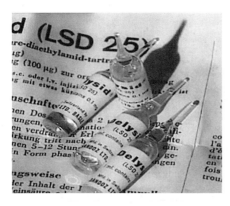

Vials of Delysid, marketed by the pharmaceutical company Sandoz, which contained a dilution of LSD-25. Photo sourced from "El primer estudio sobre el LSD en 40 años le vuelve a encontrar potencial terapéutico" [The first study on LSD in 40 years once again finds therapeutic potential] by Nico Varonas via the Neoteo website.

the last months of their life. Fortunately, other groups were also able to study and later replicate this approach, to the point that treating death depression with psychedelic psychotherapy ended up being reproduced with good results in contexts in which death was not the evident cause of depression, and it kept evolving until becoming a useful therapy in depression not associated with death.

Cohen would end up becoming a great defender of the therapeutic potential of psychedelics, but also one of the main disseminators of the dangers of using it outside the clinic, publishing articles on the risks of misused psychedelics.

But scientists, doctors, and intellectuals were not the only parties interested in harnessing the power of psychedelics. Between 1953 and 1973, the CIA carried out the secret project MKUltra (acronym for *mind control ultra*) performing illegal human experimentation, which sought to find substances and techniques that would facilitate interrogations, brainwashing, mind control, torture, and to explore their potential military use.[15] In the context of this secret project, multiple inhuman experiments were carried out with psychedelic, depressant, and deliriant drugs,[16] among other techniques, on volunteers or even civilians without their knowledge or consent. In some cases, these experiments ended in tragedy.

---

15. Martin A. Lee and Bruce Shlain, *Acid Dreams: The Complete Social History of LSD: The CIA, the Sixties, and Beyond* (New York: Grove Atlantic, 1992).
16. Category of substances that, unlike most psychedelics, induce delirium. They normally have an anticholinergic effect on the brain.

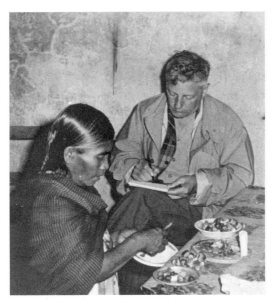

María Sabina prepares psilocybe mushrooms while Robert G. Wasson
takes notes. Photo from Robert Gordon Wasson,
"Seeking the Magic Mushroom," *Life*, May 13, 1957.

In 1955, the American banker and ethnobotanist Robert Gordon
Wasson and his wife, pediatrician and researcher Valentina Wasson,
were inspired by an article by the ethnobotanist Richard Evans Schultes
and traveled to Mexico to participate in a Mazatec ritual with psilocybe mushrooms, invited by *curandera* (healer) María Sabina. Upon
his return, Gordon published an article in the popular magazine *Life*
titled "Seeking the Magic Mushroom"[17] in 1957. They also accompanied the French mycologist Roger Heim to take samples, which he
would later cultivate in France and send to Albert Hofmann for study,
with the suspicion that it might contain a substance similar to LSD.
After carrying out another first-person experiment with mushrooms,
realizing their similarity to LSD, Albert Hofmann isolated, synthesized, and described their active ingredients: psilocybin and psilocin,
psychedelic tryptamines very similar to LSD at the structural and
pharmacological level, although with different pharmacokinetics and

17. Robert Gordon Wasson, "Seeking the Magic Mushroom," *Life* (May 13, 1957).

less pharmacological potency and duration of effects. Sandoz began marketing psilocybin under the trade name Indocybin with similar indications as LSD. At this point in history, Albert Hofmann had already become a scientist whose career would be marked by the various psychedelic tryptamines that he himself discovered and described for Western science, convinced of their scientific and therapeutic usefulness, but which would suffer severe legislative setbacks yet to come.

In the late 1950s, LSD was already very popular in psychiatry. Some psychoanalysts at the time considered that LSD allowed them to reach depths inaccessible to traditional therapeutic methods, and much more quickly, saving years of therapy. Sometimes therapists even took LSD with their patients to facilitate empathic bonds. In 1959 psychiatrist Duncan Blewett, along with Alfred Hubbard and Humphry Osmond, published the *Handbook for the Therapeutic Use of LSD*,[18] considered one of the best guides to the clinical use of this substance. Blewett himself was so convinced that his approach was working above all other therapy that he considered LSD psychotherapy to produce better results in a single afternoon than several years of conventional therapy.

Some personalities of the time had the opportunity to access these new psychedelic psychotherapy treatments with very positive results, such as the wife of then U.S. Senator Robert Kennedy (who would later defend the medical potential of LSD before its imminent prohibition) or the famous actor Cary Grant, who declared that he felt like a man "reborn" after several sessions of LSD. These experiences were widely aired by the media and gave a certain glamor to these new experiences. Unfortunately, however, results were not always so positive and there were those who, outside of adequately controlled clinical use, sometimes had negative experiences. Although these cases rarely had lasting results, they were juicy enough for the most puritanical tabloid press.

By the early 1960s, LSD's popularity had moved out of scientific and therapeutic circles and onto the streets, where it was being used without medical supervision for recreational, spiritual, social, political, cultural,

---

18. N. Chwelos and D. B. Blewett, "Handbook for the Therapeutic Use of Lysergic Acid Diehylamide 25: Individual and Group Procedures," (no publisher, 1959).

and self-exploration purposes. They were closely associated with youth counterculture movements, such as the hippie movement, with input from Beat Generation artists and writers such as William Burroughs, Allen Ginsberg, and many others who were beginning to experiment with LSD. In California, a group of young people calling themselves "The Merry Pranksters," formed by some famous names from the world of the arts such as the writer Ken Kesey, who had been a volunteer for the MKUltra project, began to tour the country giving LSD to people as a rite of passage known as "acid test," and greatly popularizing its use at the street level. It was precisely at this time that the first problems for LSD began, with the popularization of its use outside of controlled research settings.

Echoes of this countercultural movement reached Harvard in 1962, where Professor Timothy Leary was very interested in the use of psychedelics since he had had experiences with psilocybin mushrooms—even claiming that he had learned more about psychology in five hours with them than in his fifteen years of research. He began to conduct first-person experiments, organize studies together with his colleagues Ralph Metzner and Richard Alpert (later known as Ram Dass), and to include them in his classes with his students in what is known as the Harvard

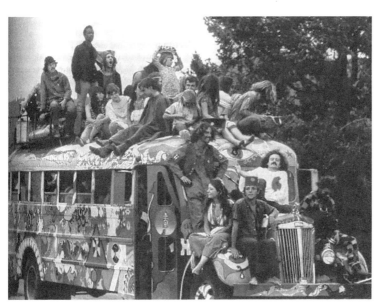

The Merry Pranksters bus on tour in the United States with their acid test. Photo by Scott Brenner, "The Merry Pranksters," via The American Century website.

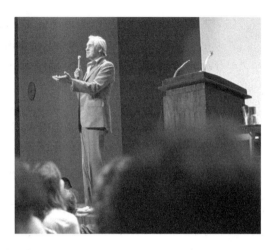

Timothy Leary, speaking at Southern Illinois University at Carbondale. Photo by Brian Crawford.

Psilocybin Project, which consisted of several experiments with psilocybin in class, prisons, and even the famous "Good Friday" experiment[19] (or Marsh Chapel Experiment), conducted by a graduate student under Leary named Walter Pahnke, in which several theology students (among them the later famous Huston Smith) received psilocybin to attend mass and study whether it produced a mystical experience in them, which it did, in all of them, as opposed to those who only received a placebo. After growing concerns about Leary and Alpert's controversial work and the administration of psychedelic drugs to undergraduate students, Harvard University decided to fire them in 1963.

After his dismissal from Harvard, Leary moved to a country house in Millbrook where he founded a psychedelic commune, in which many young people came together and which served as the first great experiment in the social consumption of psychedelics for "psychological and spiritual development." This place served as a loudspeaker for the model that they intended to export to the entire American society, advocating that youth abandon their studies and join the movement, an invitation that years later would spread using the slogan "Turn on, tune in, drop out." One of the regulars at Millbrook was Mary Pinchot (lover of President John F. Kennedy) who, together with Leary, planned to initiate

---

19. Walter Norman Pahnke, *Drugs and Mysticism: An Analysis of the Relationship between Psychedelic Drugs and the Mystical Consciousness: A Thesis* (Cambridge, MA, Harvard University, 1963).

different political personalities in the use of psychedelics and thus reduce the military tensions of the cold war. It has always been speculated that President John F. Kennedy himself may have experienced an LSD or psilocybin trip facilitated by Pinchot.

From Millbrook, Albert Hofmann and Sandoz received a request for a large quantity of LSD and psilocybin, which they rejected, stating these substances were still in the research phase and that they disapproved of the uncontrolled use of psychedelic tryptamines taking place at the commune. Albert Hofmann refused to take part in that movement and accused them of discrediting all the scientific work that was being done at that time, putting it at risk. At this point, tensions gradually began to grow between the controlled research use and uncontrolled social and countercultural use of psychedelics, which would continue until their complete prohibition years later.

Most of the scientific community at the time censored what was happening at Millbrook and saw years of research with psychedelics jeopardized if their popularization outside controlled environments could not be stopped. But Sandoz's restriction of supplies did not achieve its goal. Instead of reducing the uncontrolled use of its molecules, when Millbrook's supply ran out, anthropologist Nick Sand, who was a member of the commune and had a background in chemistry, began to manufacture millions of doses. This enabled them to become self-sufficient and supply the black market, which they continued to do years later when they moved to California, even making them the main LSD supplier of the American market for many years.

Another important development of those years was the study of psychedelic substances as enhancers of creativity, associated with the field of business innovation, fundamentally applied to science and technology. A series of experiments by the research team of James Fadiman and Myron J. Stolaroff, among others, showed how low or medium doses of these substances could unlock breakthroughs or make it easier to solve technical problems.[20] In this area, the use of psychedelics as enhancers

---

20. W. W. Harman et al., "Psychedelic agents in creative problem-solving: A pilot study," *Psychological Reports* 19, no. 1 (August 1966): 211–27.

of creativity began to have many defenders within the world of science, technology, and art, a trend that has continued to this day, and that along the way has had the support of personalities such as Steve Jobs (Founder and Chairman of Apple), Francis Crick (Nobel Prize winner for his discovery of the DNA double helix), neuroscientist John C. Lilly, Kary Mullis (Nobel Prize winner for the discovery of PCR), Richard Feynman (Nobel Prize winner in physics), Oliver Sacks, Jean-Paul Sartre, Michel Foucault, and countless artists and musicians (The Beatles, Pink Floyd, The Doors, The Grateful Dead, Brian Wilson, Ray Charles, Eric Clapton, The Beach Boys, and Jimi Hendrix). Nowadays, the microdosing trend is a low-dose adaptation of the daily work of this same principle of psychedelics as creativity enhancers.

Another event that would eventually prove to be of great importance is the synthesis of ketamine in 1962 by the chemist Calvin Lee Stevens of Wayne State University who was working as a consultant for the pharmaceutical company Parke-Davis (now part of Pfizer). After passing clinical trials in prisoners, it was shown to be a much safer anesthetic with more controllable effects and a shorter duration than phencyclidine (PCP), producing "disconnection" effects that some researchers said resembled a sleep state, although they were later defined as dissociative. This substance would finally be approved as an anesthetic by the Food

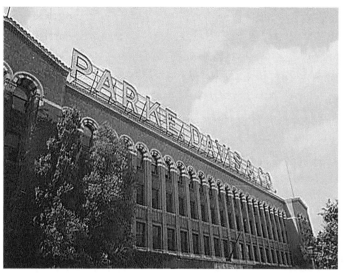

Parke-Davis Pharmaceuticals, currently part of Pfizer. Photo from the U.S. Farm Security Administration – Office of War Information photograph collection.

and Drug Administration (FDA) in 1970 and, since then, its use in medicine has been very extensive, given its efficacy and safety. Although various researchers also began to be interested in these dissociative states induced by the substance and their work would, ultimately, be of great therapeutic and recreational interest.

In the early 1960s the operation of Canadian psychedelic research was complicated by a political and managerial change at the Saskatchewan Hospital in Canada and by Abram Hoffer's confrontation with conventional psychiatry (which feared the excessive popularization of the still novel psychedelic psychotherapy), and by the appearance of information in the media linking LSD to chromosome damage, defects in fetuses, cancer, accidents, and cases of psychosis and suicides. Years later it was demonstrated that much of this news was untrue, and that the cases of psychosis were mostly the product of failures in the administration of LSD, using unsuitable subjects (who should have been dismissed), or without adequate preparation. In addition, clinical suicide rates were proven to be even lower than those of conventional therapies. Still, the damage to political and public opinion on psychedelics had already been done.

Some meta-analyses and questionnaires were conducted to study the safety and risks of psychedelic-assisted psychotherapy, especially using LSD and psilocybin. In the United States it was Dr. Sidney Cohen, psychiatrist and professor at the University of California in Los Angeles, who published in this regard in 1960; in England it was the psychiatrist of the Royal Society, Dr. Nicolas Malleson. The results of the studies (with 25,000 observations in the case of Cohen and 49,500 in the Malleson study) showed a very low hazard level of these substances in controlled psychotherapeutic settings (despite the fact that the psychedelic technique was not yet fully optimized), which did not correspond with the discourse of danger that was increasingly being offered by governments and the media.

In 1963, at Spring Grove Hospital, the U.S. National Institute of Mental Health (NIMH) financed a study of LSD-assisted psychotherapy in alcoholics, which confirmed the good results that this type of therapy offered, achieving great visibility with the broadcast of a report

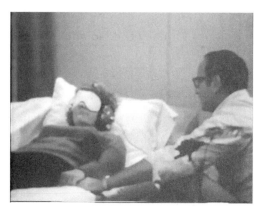

Sanford Unger, a researcher at Spring Grove, with a patient in an LSD psychotherapy session. Photo from "LSD: The Spring Grove Experiment," CBS Reports, produced by John Sharnik and Harry Morgan, aired May 17, 1966, *CBS News Archives*, 2016, DVD.

on the CBS television network. This study also allowed for an improvement in the technique by giving value to factors that had previously been little attended to, such as the patient's physical environment and their mental state at the time of taking the psychedelic, what came to be known as "set and setting," for which an adequate prior screening was vital to guarantee that the patients who accessed the treatment were in a position to benefit from it as much as possible, minimizing the risks.

Despite all these developments, in 1963 in Canada a series of very notorious negative events related to the recreational use of LSD in young people prompted the country's new government to impose strict control measures on the substance, which would seriously hinder research and lead many of its researchers to abandon their work (as was the case with the Saskatchewan Hospital group) and would contribute to the growth of a black market for the substance, which, in turn, was accompanied by a greater number of public health problems in the country.

In the mid-1960s, after the publication of the manual *The Psychedelic Experience: A Manual Based on the Tibetan Book of the Dead*[21] and the continuous growth of the hippie culture and the pacifist movement against the Vietnam War, San Francisco began to bring together a large number of young people who came from all over the country and whose poorly controlled use of psychedelic substances began to increase the incidence of problems related to them. The consumption

21. Timothy Leary, Ralph Metzner, and Richard Alpert, *The Psychedelic Experience: A Manual Based on the Tibetan Book of the Dead* (University Books, 1964).

of psychedelics was beginning to be considered a problem of public order, not only because of its implications for daily functioning in cities but also because of the changes in political, ethical, and cultural values to which it was linked. Particularly relevant was the rebellious nature of the pacifist and civil rights movements, strengthened by the experiences of unity and empathy that were associated with the psychedelic experience in a propitious context such as that of the Vietnam War, to which thousands of young people were sent against their will—all this mixed with a potentially destabilizing countercultural revolution and a questioning of the moral legitimacy of the authorities. It would be very risky to say that psychedelics were the cause of these social changes, but it is undeniable that they were associated with them, if only because of their repeated use by their promoters and members, and they became a symbol of the movement. In this context, public administrations and the press began to project a very distorted image of psychedelics, associating them with everything that was wrong—suicides, murders, malformations, accidents, rapes, cults—and disseminating large dissuasive advertising campaigns about their consumption, unleashing a panic that joined the already existing one in the most puritanical sectors of the United States.

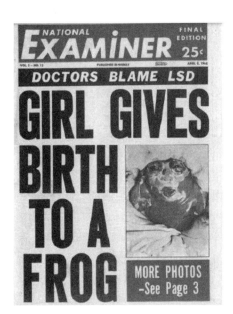

"Woman Gives Birth to Frog, Doctors Blame LSD." The media spread much sensational fake news against psychedelics.

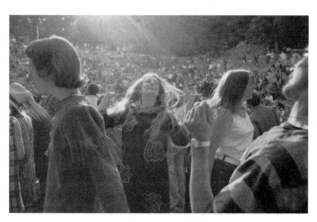

Thousands of young people gathered in San Francisco in the summer of 1967,
"The Summer of Love." Photo by Elaine Mayes. Fantasy Fair, Mill Valley, 1967.
Featured in *On the Road to the Summer of Love*,
an exhibition at the California Historical Society.

In 1966, at a congressional subcommittee evaluating the restriction
of psychedelics chaired by Senator Robert Kennedy, who was opposed
to its complete prohibition, he declared:

> Why if [clinical LSD projects] were worthwhile six months ago, why
> aren't they worthwhile now? I think we have given too much empha-
> sis and so much attention to the fact that [LSD] can be dangerous
> and that it can hurt an individual who uses it that perhaps to some
> extent we have lost sight of the fact that it can be very, very helpful
> in our society if used properly.[22]

In October 1966, the state of California decided to ban LSD for
all uses. In the eyes of the administration, condemning the possession
and use of psychedelics was not only a way of showing the electorate
their commitment to preserving health, morals, and public order, but
it was also a way of being able to take legal action against members of
a social movement that was becoming extremely uncomfortable for the
government at the time. This ban led to demonstrations and riots in

---

22. Martin A. Lee and Bruce Shlain, *Acid Dreams: The Complete Social History of LSD:
The CIA, The Sixties, and Beyond* (New York: Grove Press, 1985); see page 78.

the United States, like the famous protest at the Golden Gate Park in San Francisco, where twenty thousand people gathered to consume psychedelics. Nor did this legislation prevent the phenomenon from continuing to grow in that city, especially in the Haight-Ashbury neighborhood, giving rise to what was known as the "Summer of Love" in 1967, one of the landmark moments of the hippie movement, but further evidence of the lack of control that was being practiced in the use of these substances outside clinics and laboratories.

The expiration of the Sandoz Delysid patent was seen as an appropriate occasion to abandon the manufacture and sale of LSD, given the perception of great social turmoil offered by the press in the United States and Canada, blaming it on the use of the substance, and how badly this reflected on Sandoz; although its clinical use continued to be very promising and its controlled use did not seem to be causing any relevant problems, on the street the perception was very different. Unfortunately, some researchers with access to the substance did not want to limit it to strictly clinical use, which justified much broader restrictions than would have been expected and led to its definitive ban for all uses.

In 1968, coinciding with student revolts in Europe and the United States, LSD was definitively banned throughout the whole U.S. territory, which was a blow to the research that was in progress and forced promising ongoing studies, as well as its therapeutic use, to stop. But the main objective of curbing the use of LSD in society was not achieved, since a powerful black market had developed that would continue to supply the public from then until today. As proof of the United States' perception of the lack of control that had been reached in the recreational use of psychedelics and the social impact of the counterculture of the time, Richard Nixon, president of the United States, commenced a smear campaign against all uses of LSD and psychedelics (including scientific), and years later apparently declared Timothy Leary "the most dangerous man in America."

This total prohibition movement did not mean the disappearance of LSD or psilocybin from the streets, since there was already a vast production and distribution network that was not only well supplied and very

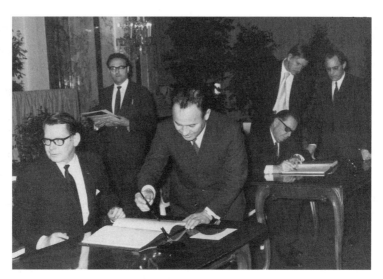

Signing of the United Nations Convention on Psychotropic Substances of 1971.

profitable (one gram of LSD gives about ten thousand doses, and mushrooms with psilocybin are easy and cheap to grow at home), but in many cases, this network claimed to have more political and even philanthropic purposes than economic (as in the case of the Brotherhood of Eternal Love), given that psychedelics had become the fuel of the counterculture and the hippie movement. The frequent confiscation of millions of doses did not reduce access to the substance; however, this movement did mean the end of all scientific and clinical research, which was so difficult and expensive that it became blocked de facto and had to be abandoned.

In 1971, the U.S. president Richard Nixon stated that drugs were "public enemy number one" and declared a "war on drugs," a global campaign aimed at eradicating drugs through the use of all available legislative, police, economic, and military instruments. That same year, with the strong influence of the United States, the United Nations Convention on Psychotropic Substances was signed in Vienna.[23] It imposed four lists or schedules for classifying controlled psychoactive substances, correspond-

---

23. The term psychotropic refers to substances that modify the mind, such as LSD, psilocybin and MDMA. The 1971 UN Convention on Psychotropic Substances focused on controlling them internationally based on their potential for abuse or risk.

ing to four different levels of international control, where these substances were no longer only controlled because of their risk of addiction (as was the case of the 1961 convention on narcotic substances[24]) but because of their mind-altering ability, alleged potential for abuse, and risk to public health. These restrictions included their authorized medical uses, regardless of their addictiveness (most classic psychedelics are not addictive). Psychedelics (LSD, psilocybin, mescaline and DMT) were placed on the most controlled list, Schedule I, reserved for substances "with great potential risk to public health and no recognized medical use."

MDMA

3,4-methylenedioxymethamphetamine (MDMA, also known today as ecstasy) was synthesized for the first time in 1912 by the German chemist Anton Köllisch for the pharmaceutical company Merck (and patented by them, as well) as an intermediate compound for the synthesis of a hemostatic agent,[25] but this substance didn't get attention at the time. It wasn't until the 1950s that it began to spark some interest, and it is said that the U.S. military performed some studies with it, among other psychoactive substances, in the context of their MKUltra project. In 1965, Alexander "Sasha" Shulguin, a biochemist who worked for Dow Chemical, synthesized this compound. In the 1970s, after the prohibition of MDA (a drug similar in molecular structure and effects, which had become popular), cases of recreational use of MDMA began to appear in the Chicago area.

In 1976, after talking to Merrie Kleinman, a student who had tried MDMA, Alexander Shulgin decided to try it and was deeply impressed by the effects of this substance on the emotional level and its therapeutic potential. He later shared several of these MDMA experiences with his partner Ann and some close friends and published, together with biochemist David E. Nichols, the first scientific

---

24. The term narcotic refers to substances that stimulate or depress the CNS, such as morphine or cocaine. The 1961 UN Single Convention on Narcotic Drugs focused on controlling drugs internationally based on their risk of addiction.

25. A hemostatic agent is a substance that facilitates blood coagulation and thus stops bleeding.

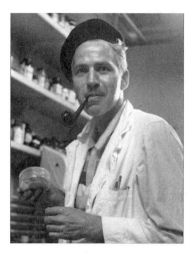

Alexander "Sasha" Shulgin, rediscoverer and "godfather" of MDMA, and discoverer of hundreds of new psychedelic molecules.
Photo sourced via the Erowid website.

article on MDMA's effects on humans, describing them as "an easily controllable altered state of consciousness with emotional and sensual overtones," comparable to "marijuana, psilocybin devoid of its hallucinatory component, or low levels of MDA."[26]

Sensing that its effects could be of enormous help for psychotherapy, he showed it to psychotherapist Leo Zeff, who was impressed by its potential and introduced it to the circles of psychotherapists and psychiatrists, teaching thousands of professionals to work with the substance. He nicknamed it "Adam," alluding to its ability to put people in states of "primordial innocence." MDMA was used in combination with psychotherapy, improving the capacity for introspection, work on the traumatic past, therapist-patient connection, and was able to accelerate the treatment of diseases such as post-traumatic stress disorder, depression, addictions, and even couple conflicts, thanks to its ability to induce empathy, positive emotions, improve communication and facilitate forgiveness, because, among other things, MDMA "does not open the doors of perception [like classic psychedelics] as much as of emotionality."[27]

26. Alexander T. Shulgin and David E. Nichols, "Characterization of Three New Psychotomimetics," in *The Psychopharmacology of Hallucinogens*, ed. Richard C. Stillman and Robert E. Willette (Amsterdam: Elsevier, 1978), 74–83.
27. Antonio Escohotado, *Historia Elemental de las Drogas* [The General History of Drugs] (Barcelona: Anagrama, 2006).

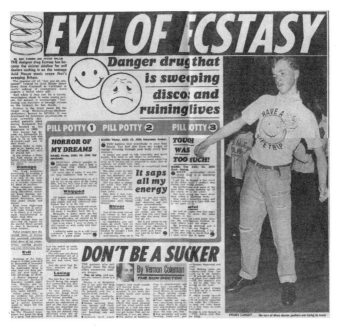

"The evil of ecstasy. The dangerous drug that is sweeping nightclubs and ruining lives. A nightmare. Don't be a fool." As with LSD and other psychedelics, MDMA also had its own campaign of sensationalism.

Although MDMA was known as "empathy" or "Adam," the press preferred to popularize the term "ecstasy" (also "XTC" or "X"), coined in relation to the effects of its recreational use. Its recreational heyday came in the mid-1980s, with the new age movement and the rave scene; and, just as it had happened with psychedelics, based on negative reports and some deaths from heat stroke or overdose, the media began to publish highly exaggerated, sensational, and even fake news about the substance and what happened in the raves among the young people who consumed it, initiating a moral panic that would quickly spread.

In 1985, the U.S. Drug Enforcement Administration (DEA) urgently banned MDMA for all uses, despite the fact that many therapists and psychiatrists testified against this ban citing the "almost incredible capacity of MDMA to facilitate subjective communication and access to repressed feelings," arguments that were not taken into account when the substance was also prohibited for clinical use and research.

Soon after, the expert committee of the World Health Organization (WHO) concluded that:

No data are available concerning its clinical abuse liability, nature and magnitude of associated public health or social problems, or epidemiology of its use and abuse. . . . The substance has no well defined therapeutic use; but a number of clinicians in the USA have claimed that it is potentially valuable as a psychotherapeutic agent. . . . It should be noted that the Expert Committee held extensive discussions concerning the reported therapeutic usefulness of 3,4-methylenedioxymethamphetamine. While the Expert Committee found the reports intriguing, it felt that the studies lacked the appropriate methodological design necessary to ascertain the reliability of the observations. There was, however, sufficient interest expressed to recommend that investigations be encouraged to follow up these preliminary findings. To that end, the Expert Committee urged countries to use the provisions of article 7 of the Convention on Psychotropic Substances to facilitate research on this interesting substance. [One member, Professor Paul Grof (Chairman), felt that the decision on the recommendation should be deferred awaiting, in particular, the data on the substance's potential therapeutic usefulness and that at this time international control is not warranted.][28]

Despite all this, it was included in Schedule I of the Convention on Psychotropic Substances of the United Nations as a substance "with a great potential risk to public health and no recognized medical use," dashing any hope of further use by the medical and research communities.

In 1986, the year after the prohibition of MDMA, which was the last great promise in the field of psychedelics with clinical potential, Rick Doblin founded the Multidisciplinary Association for the Study

---

28. World Health Organization, *WHO Expert Committee on Drug Dependence: Twenty-Second Report*, WHO Technical Report Series No. 729, 1985; see page 25.

of Psychedelics (MAPS), a nonprofit scientific-advocacy organization, to continue promoting rigorous scientific research into the therapeutic use of psychedelics and appeal to the necessary legal channels to return these substances to clinics, laboratories, and a future society that knows how to use them with responsibility and discretion.

AFTER THE BAN

Despite the fact that, by the mid-1960s, the clinical use of psychedelics had already led to the publication of dozens of books and the organization of several international conferences, in addition to the publication of more than one thousand peer-reviewed scientific articles in which these substances had been administered to more than forty thousand participants,[29] research in psychotherapy with LSD and psilocybin failed to take root. Initially, it was due to the fact that the science used in the 1950s, mainly at the Saskatchewan Hospital, did not meet all the scientific standards that would be required years later, nor was it as methodical or controlled as it should have been to give the irrefutable results that would leave a greater mark on the world of psychiatry.[30] The effects of these substances were also more difficult to predict in those early years, something that was uncomfortable to manage in the clinic.

However, starting in the 1960s, when LSD's application, safety, and predictability seemed to improve, its great failure was not having been able to detach itself from the sociopolitical context and thus prevent the popularization of the use of LSD on the streets, with former researchers promoting its massive use, and their inevitable association with the counterculture, student protests, peace movements, and movements against Vietnam, which ended up polarizing the position of governments that would end up banning psychedelics; and with them, any legitimate use of these (until then) promising substances for research purposes. Also,

29. L. Grinspoon and J. B. Bakalar, "The Psychedelic Drug Therapies," *Current Psychiatric Therapies* 20 (1981): 275–83.

30. Erika Dyck, "Flashback: Psychiatric Experimentation with LSD in Historical Perspective," *Canadian Journal of Psychiatry* 50, no. 7 (June 2005): 381–88.

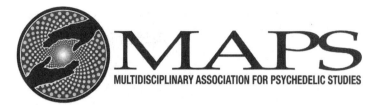

Logo of the Multidisciplinary Association for the Study of Psychedelics, founded by Rick Doblin in 1986 after the prohibition of MDMA.

changes in clinical research related to the thalidomide scandal[31] made these substances more difficult to research and new developments in psychopharmacological treatments greatly diminished pharmaceutical interest in psychedelics, while stigma did the rest to deter researchers from getting into the field or continuing research on it.

With the exception of ketamine, the history of the classic psychedelics (psilocybin, LSD, mescaline) and that of MDMA had followed a similar script: substances with promising scientific and medical use, but which were banned when they became popular outside of clinics and laboratories, becoming a scapegoat to control certain youth or political movements. Their risks and harms outside of clinical use were real, but were taken out of context and exaggerated considering the enormous harms of alcohol, tobacco, and other legal substances. Unfortunately, the ban was only effective in crippling scientific research and the clinical use of these substances because, as is the case with almost all drugs, the ban did not have the expected effect on their recreational or non-supervised use. Quite the opposite, their popularity in these contexts continued to grow, counting the doses consumed and confiscated around the world each year in the millions. All this resulted in an even less informed use due to taboo, an increase in the adulteration of the substance, and therefore, an increase in physical and mental health risks.

---

31. The thalidomide scandal occurred in the late 1950s and early 1960s when the drug thalidomide, marketed as a treatment for morning sickness in pregnant women, caused severe birth defects in thousands of babies worldwide. The drug, which was not initially tested for use during pregnancy, led to babies being born with limb deformities, such as shortened or absent arms and legs, as well as other severe health issues. The scandal led to stricter drug regulations and testing requirements globally.

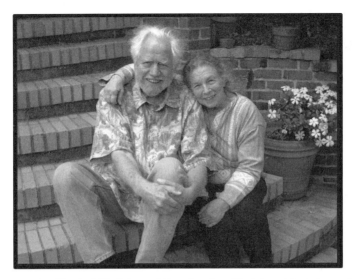

Alexander "Sasha" Shulgin and his wife, Ann Shulgin, at their home in
Lafayette, California, 2002. Photo by Anthony Pidgeon/Redferns.

Despite the ban, unofficial research into psychedelics and underground treatments continued in the following decades, with psychedelic-
assisted psychotherapies sometimes using other non-illegalized
psychedelic compounds or other non-pharmacological techniques to
access altered states of consciousness, such as holotropic breathwork.
Given the illegal nature of many of these investigations and treatments,
there were few publications about them, but some people dared to do
so, such as George Greer, Myron Stolaroff, Athanasios Kafkalides, and
the Shulgins.

Biochemist Alexander "Sasha" Shulgin and his wife, Ann Shulgin,
who had extensively researched the chemistry and effects of different
psychedelics on the body, especially MDMA, feeling that these pharmacological tools had been unfairly banned for reasons unrelated to
science, decided to share their knowledge to encourage research and
self-exploration by publishing in 1991 the book *PiHKAL: A Chemical
Love Story*[32] (the acronym stands for Phenethylamines I Have Known

---

32. Alexander Theodore Shulgin and Ann Shulgin, *PiHKAL: A Chemical Love Story*
(Berkeley: Transform Press, 1991).

and Loved), and in the book they tell their own story with 179 substances from this chemical family (which includes psychedelics such as
mescaline, and empathogens/entactogens with psychedelic properties
such as MDMA), most of them discovered by Shulgin, as well as the
recipes to synthesize them, dosages, and laboratory notes.

The DEA (Drug Enforcement Administration) was angry with the
chemist after finding his book being used by several illicit drug laboratories and decided to raid and close his laboratory in 1994, revoking his
license to investigate and produce illegalized drugs.

In response to this, the couple was reinforced in their conviction
to prevent these substances from falling into scientific oblivion, and
in 1997 they published the book *TiHKAL: The Continuation*.[33] The
acronym stands for Tryptamines I Have Known and Loved, and this
book followed a very similar structure to the previous one, but this time
focused on their experiences with fifty-five molecules of the chemical
family of tryptamines (to which most classic psychedelics belong, such
as psilocybin, psilocin, LSD, and DMT).

---

33. Alexander Theodore Shulgin and Ann Shulgin, *TiHKAL: The Continuation*
(Berkeley: Transform Press, 1997).

4

The Psychedelic Renaissance

As we saw in the previous chapter, although natural psychedelics from plants, fungi, and animals had been used in some cultures for millennia, it was Albert Hofmann's discovery of LSD back in 1943 that really started and spurred the interest and research of these substances in the West. This scientific interest and research in psychedelics greatly advanced the study of the brain, as well as helped to lay the foundations for the relationship between neurochemistry and behavior, allowing the development of very promising new models of experimental treatments in mental health using these substances, such as psychedelic-assisted psychotherapies. With these new treatment models, it was possible, for example, for people suffering from terminal cancer to recover their smile in their last months of life, or for people suffering from alcoholism to stop drinking.[1] But this whole movement became deadlocked due to various factors: psychedelics' use (outside the clinic or the laboratory) by counterculture and anti-Vietnam war movements (which made the U.S. government and various conservative sectors very uncomfortable), some over-sensationalized cases by the press, the ignorance surrounding psychedelics' neurological functioning and long-term consequences, plus the various campaigns in the media[2] along with a diminished interest

---

1. Teri S. Krebs and Pål-Ørjan Johansen, "Lysergic Acid Diethylamide (LSD) for Alcoholism: Meta-Analysis of Randomized Controlled Trials," *Journal of Psychopharmacology* 26, no. 7 (July 2012): 994–1002.
2. Stephen Siff, *Acid Hype: American News Media and the Psychedelic Experience* (Champaign, University of Illinois Press, 2015).

by the pharmaceutical industry in psychedelic research and development. All these led the U.S. government at the time to ban them at the federal level in 1968 and, soon after, psychedelics were also controlled internationally. Thus began the famous "war on drugs," ending a prolific era of very promising clinical research. Years later, history would repeat itself with MDMA (ecstasy) using a very similar script, destroying a substance with enormous clinical potential after its prohibition in 1985, despite the opposition of a good part of the scientific community and its "sponsorship" by Alexander "Sasha" Shulgin and Ann Shulguin.

This could have been the end of the story. Psychedelics would be just another family of illegalized drugs with supposedly "great potential risk to public health and no recognized medical use" as the United Nations says—a marginal family of substances doomed to oblivion and within the reach of only a few avid psychonauts. It would have stayed this way if it had not been for the determination and tenacity of some people and organizations that, despite the legal difficulties imposed, maintained the conviction that psychedelics had enormous potential and could have an important place in our society if they were used and controlled properly.

Nowadays there is a lot of talk about psychedelics everywhere: studies of magic mushrooms to treat all kinds of disorders, such as depression and addictions; celebrities doing ayahuasca retreats; LSD microdosing to improve productivity in Silicon Valley startups; MDMA (ecstasy) being a few steps away from becoming legalized by the FDA to cure traumas and meetings on future regulations on and implementations of MDMA and other psychedelics already taking place at the European Medicines Agency; ketamine administered to billionaires and celebrities in overpriced mental health clinics; debates in the European Parliament and the U.S. Congress, where there are initiatives and talks of lowering the legal control of psychedelics; prestigious universities creating psychedelic research centers and psychedelic training curriculums; reputable scientific journals naming psychedelic therapies among the year's greatest scientific breakthroughs; "psychedelic" companies trading on Wall Street and receiving billions of dollars in investments; U.S. cities and states decriminalizing or even legalizing the possession and use of psychedelics;

books on the subject becoming bestsellers; podcasts with millions of listeners where celebrity guests share their psychedelic journeys; psychedelic music festivals among the most famous in the world; series on Netflix on the subject and many articles in all kinds of media. Without going any further, a few years ago the *New York Times* ran the following headline on its cover to summarize the phenomenon in the scientific field: "The Psychedelic Revolution Is Coming. Psychiatry May Never Be the Same."[3]

What's going on? Weren't these substances supposed to be dangerous drugs with no medical use? Why is this happening now?

ONGOING PSYCHEDELICS RESEARCH

Although the official story of "dangerous drugs with no medical use" spread by governments and the press, together with legal restrictions, worked well as a deterrent at a scientific level for decades, relegating these substances almost to oblivion (in contrast with their recreational use, which continued to be very popular), since the end of the twentieth century and especially in the beginning of the twenty-first century, some researchers, thanks to their conviction, and despite the great bureaucratic challenges, resumed official lines of research related to psychedelics.

Some were veterans of the research conducted in the 1950s, 1960s, and 1970s, and others had held parallel lines to psychedelics, while brave newcomers also joined the field.

This time, their seeds fell on fertile ground because at the beginning of this millennium numerous factors that had precipitated the prohibition of psychedelic substances in the late 1960s were changing, and many others appeared, facilitating the conditions for lines of research with psychedelics to be resumed with due caution:

- In the sociopolitical context, there had been a stabilization with respect to the years in which its prohibition originated: appeasement

---

3. Andrew Jacobs, "The Psychedelic Revolution Is Coming. Psychiatry May Never Be the Same," *New York Times*, May 9, 2021.

of the student revolts and the pacifist movement; end of the political tension of the cold war; end of the antinuclear movement and no more wars that required forced recruitment. In short, the sociocultural context that had used psychedelics as an identity element of rebellion against the government was already extinct, as was the generation of politicians who had confronted them.

- In the epidemiological context, where mental illnesses such as depression, anxiety, post-traumatic stress disorder, addictions, or neurodegenerative disorders are a growing major problem, especially in Western societies (and even more so after the COVID-19 pandemic), it is becoming increasingly urgent to innovate and accelerate the progress of neuroscience to understand the pathological mechanisms of these diseases, as well as to search for new and better treatments.

- Together with the above, there is an urgent need for new advances in treatments and psychopharmacology, which has been quite stagnant for decades, and has not made great progress since the discovery of antidepressants that inhibit the reuptake of different types of neurotransmitters (SSRIs and SNRIs such as fluoxetine [Prozac] and venlafaxine [Effexor]) and benzodiazepines (such as alprazolam [Xanax]).

- In the context of scientific research, the development of neuroscience and neurochemistry, together with the development of neuroimaging techniques (such as positron emission tomography, PET, and magnetic resonance imaging or MRIs), has facilitated the work, allowing a better theoretical understanding and practical observation of the mechanisms of action of psychedelic substances, and with it, improvements in the predictability and control of their risks, opening the way to apply their therapeutic and research potential, as well as the communication of said findings.

- The improvement of scientific standards, research designs, and analytic tools, which make the results more solid and undeniable, in addition to establishing correlations and causalities more easily.

- Many of the researchers involved in the research of the 1950s and 1960s (although some were already at the end of their careers) were still close to the field and maintained their interest and conviction that these substances had a great role to play in modern science, having been able to lead or support the resurgence with their expertise and knowledge.

- In addition, a new generation of unprejudiced researchers is emerging, wanting to innovate and advance the field of neuroscience and therapy, challenging the taboos on substances that proved not to be as dangerous or as useless as they were labeled, but rather have great potential.

- The growing number and support of scientific institutions specialized in psychedelic research such as the Multidisciplinary Association for Psychedelic Studies (MAPS), the Heffter Research Institute, the Beckley Foundation, the International Center for Ethnobotanical Education, Research, and Service (ICEERS), and many more, together with a greater openness and acceptance toward psychedelic research by teams and ethics committees of several prestigious research organizations and centers, such as Johns Hopkins University, New York University (NYU), Harbor-UCLA Medical Center, University of New Mexico, Imperial College London, Psychiatric University Hospital of Zurich, the Hospital Sant Pau of Barcelona, and many others.

- The appearance of the internet and new communication technologies allowed information on this type of substance and its effects to circulate with greater freedom, speed, and scope, without necessarily being subject to the moral scrutiny of the mass media, thus also favoring its demystification and scientific reevaluation, as well as the dissemination of these past and present lines of research.

- Closely linked to the above, the internet also facilitated the creation of networks of people interested in the subject, as well as the accumulation of anecdotal evidence with the creation of online communities dedicated to psychonautics and the discussion of information on all kinds of psychoactive substances, such as Erowid, Reddit, Drugs-Forum, Bluelight, Cannabiscafe, and others, set up by psychonauts interested in greater knowledge and self-experimentation, and whose publications are currently analyzed by various scientific publications[4] that seek to take advantage of the experiences of these users to improve the predictability and safety of their use in clinical research. Likewise, the development of risk and harm reduction programs in recreational spaces has also made it possible to provide and validate information on how to safely manage bad experiences that may occur in clinical environments, such as, for example, the importance of set and setting or how to manage bad trips in the clinical settings. Also, the accumulation of more anecdotal evidence given its underground use.

- The review of the research carried out in the 1950s and 1960s using current standards, preparing systematic reviews and meta-analyses that have made it possible to reassess the safety and efficacy of treatments using modern tools and standards, but based on the research carried out at the time that produced many scientific publications.

- The recent acceptance of the possible medical uses of cannabis, which, in most legislation, was at the same level of prohibition as psychedelics, as in the case of the United States, where they were labeled as Schedule I substances, officially defined as being "of great risk to public health and with no therapeutic value." This acceptance also paved the way for the scientific and social acceptance of the investigation of other illegal substances, by casting doubt on the validity of old legal classifications of drugs.

- Modern population studies[5] with sample sizes in the hundreds of thousands of people, showing that there is no correlation between the use of MDMA or psychedelics and mental illness of any kind.[6] In fact, the correlation indicates that the use of MDMA or psychedelics is associated with better mental health, less

---

4. Theresa M. Carbonaro et al., "Survey Study of Challenging Experiences after Ingesting Psilocybin Mushrooms: Acute and Enduring Positive and Negative Consequences," *Journal of Psychopharmacology* 30, no. 12 (December 2016): 1268–78.

5. Teri S. Krebs and Pål-Ørjan Johansen, "Psychedelics and Mental Health: A Population Study," *PLoS One* 8, no. 8 (August 2013): e63972.

6. Pål-Ørjan Johansen and Teri Suzanne Krebs, "Psychedelics not Linked to Mental Health Problems or Suicidal Behavior: A Population Study," *Journal of Psychopharmacology* 29, no. 3 (March 2015): 270–79.

stress,[7] less depression,[8] and fewer suicidal thoughts.[9] Although "correlation does not imply causation," these studies show the extent to which the image of MDMA and psychedelics as substances that cause mental illness or attract people with mental illness is distorted by the media and prevention campaigns based on fear. The risks of these substances, while real, have been greatly overestimated, and they very rarely produce lasting negative effects.[10] They don't even seem to be associated with arrests[11] or other indicators of antisocial or criminal activities that were blamed on them in the 1960s and 1970s.

Thanks to all these factors, and many others that have emerged along the way, starting in the 1990s after a few decades of scientific silence, a few research groups began to carry out some studies with psychedelics. For example, in the United States, some studies were published with MDMA (by Charles Grob's group) and DMT (by Rick Strassman), and in Europe with ayahuasca (by Jordi Riba and Manel Barbanoj), MDMA (by Magi Farré, Rafael de la Torre, and Jordi Camí), and various other psychedelic substances such as psilocybin, MDMA, ketamine, LSD (by Franz Vollenweider and Euphrosyne Gouzoulis-Mayfrank). All this despite the fact that the rest of the scientific community was still, for

7. Peter S. Hendricks et al., "Classic Psychedelic Use Is Associated with Reduced Psychological Distress and Suicidality in the United States Adult Population," *Journal of Psychopharmacology* 29, no. 3 (March 2015): 280–88.

8. Grant M. Jones and Matthew K. Nock, "Lifetime Use of MDMA/Ecstasy and Psilocybin Is Associated with Reduced Odds of Major Depressive Episodes," *Journal of Psychopharmacology* 36, no. 1 (January 2022): 57–65.

9. Grant M. Jones and Matthew K. Nock, "MDMA/Ecstasy Use and Psilocybin Use Are Associated with Lowered Odds of Psychological Distress and Suicidal Thoughts in a Sample of U.S. Adults," *Journal of Psychopharmacology*, 36, no. 1 (January 2022): 46–56.

10. Anne K. Schlag et al., "Adverse Effects of Psychedelics: From Anecdotes and Misinformation to Systematic Science," *Journal of Psychopharmacology* 36, no. 3 (March 2022): 258–72.

11. Grant M. Jones and Matthew K. Nock, "Psilocybin Use Is Associated with Lowered Odds of Crime Arrests in U.S. Adults: A Replication and Extension," *Journal of Psychopharmacology* 36, no. 1 (January 2022): 66–73.

the most part, highly influenced by the biased view of psychedelics that had spread (and continued to spread) from prohibitionist positions, and dissuaded by the ethical, legal and economic challenges to conduct research with highly controlled substances such as psychedelics.

Unfortunately, until very recently, and even today, this research has found all kinds of obstacles and difficulties to develop, in most cases for reasons unrelated to science, as it has been the case from the 1970s. For example, in Spain, a promising study[12] on the safety and efficacy of MDMA-assisted psychotherapy in women suffering from post-traumatic stress after rape, led by José Carlos Bouso (current scientific director of ICEERS), which had begun in 2000 and was the first of therapeutic MDMA worldwide, was abruptly suspended before completion due to political pressure in 2002, despite its promising preliminary results.

Ketamine was the only substance with psychedelic properties with widely recognized medical use that had never been banned, and therefore research with it was more affordable, which allowed its antidepressant properties to be demonstrated in the year 2000[13] and meant the opening of a new clinical research and development front that would advance very quickly.

But the global scientific interest in clinical research with psychedelics began to spread faster from 2006, when Roland Griffiths, a leading researcher in the field of psychopharmacology and addictions at the prestigious Johns Hopkins University in the United States, together with a veteran of psychedelic research, William "Bill" Richards, and others, published a study[14] in which they simply administered psilocybin (the main stable active ingredient in "magic mushrooms") or placebo to a group of people in a controlled environment and under direct

---

12. José Carlos Bouso et al., "MDMA-Assisted Psychotherapy Using Low Doses in a Small Sample of Women with Chronic Posttraumatic Stress Disorder," *Journal of Psychoactive Drugs* 40, no. 3 (September 2008): 225–36.

13. Robert M. Berman et al., "Antidepressant Effects of Ketamine in Depressed Patients," *Biological Psychiatry* 47, no. 4 (February 2000): 351–4.

14. R. R. Griffiths et al., "Psilocybin Can Occasion Mystical-Type Experiences Having Substantial and Sustained Personal Meaning and Spiritual Significance," *Psychopharmacology* 187, no. 3 (August 2006): 268–83, discussion 284–92.

professional supervision in order to evaluate, after the experience, what they had felt and if it had produced lasting changes in their mood. Two thirds of the people who participated in the study rated the psilocybin psychedelic experience among the five most important and meaningful experiences of their entire lives, on the same level as the birth of a first child or the death of a close family member. A third even ranked it as the most important and meaningful experience of their lives. In addition, those who participated in the study, and their relatives, friends, and partners, testified that positive and lasting changes in different aspects of the subject's personal and emotional well-being had occurred and lasted for months.

This study and the surprising results obtained, with such an apparently simple intervention, were widely publicized and had a great impact on the scientific community (among other things, because of the signatories and the institution performing the study), and little by little continued to add new publications from various centers of great scientific prestige (e.g., Johns Hopkins University, Imperial College London, NYU, UCLA), along with the work of existing teams (University of Zurich, Hospital Sant Pau, and more) and the aforementioned veteran scientific-advocacy organizations, such as MAPS (1986), Heffter Research Institute (1993), Beckley Foundation (1998), or ICEERS (2008). These organizations had been supporting and requesting more research on the therapeutic use of psychedelics for years. Since then, they have been greatly promoting the field of psychedelic research and specifically the development of psychedelic-assisted psychotherapy at a time when we are facing a true epidemic in the field of mental health, where disorders as difficult to treat as depression, anxiety, or addictions have become the leading cause of disability worldwide (and now, after the COVID-19 pandemic, these numbers will continue to grow even faster, as various studies have already shown). Unfortunately, current conventional treatments do not achieve sufficient efficacy and efficiency rates to curb this increase in mental health problems and in many cases also lead to safety problems and side effects.

In April 2008, at the age of 102, Albert Hofmann, the main person responsible for the "discovery" and popularization of psychedelics

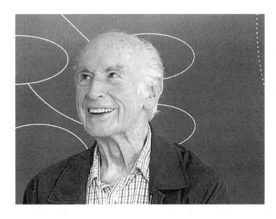

Albert Hofmann, on his 100th birthday. Photo by Stepan.

in Western science, died in Basel, Switzerland. He had always lamented that his "problematic son" (LSD) had been misinterpreted in the context of the countercultural movement, and that it had not been understood as a powerful therapeutic and spiritual tool, even declaring on his one hundredth birthday:

> It gave me an inner joy, an open mindedness, a gratefulness, open eyes and an internal sensitivity for the miracles of creation. . . . I think that in human evolution it has never been as necessary to have this substance LSD. It is just a tool to turn us into what we are supposed to be.[15]

But his death did not come without the satisfaction of seeing this psychedelic renaissance return "his" LSD to clinical research, since a year earlier, in 2007, Switzerland had authorized studies of LSD-assisted psychotherapy in terminally ill patients. These were the first studies of the therapeutic effects of LSD, conducted in humans, in thirty-five years.

Psychedelic-assisted psychotherapy is the most common form of psychedelic-assisted therapy nowadays, a treatment model in which a psychedelic is administered, in a controlled therapeutic setting, under

---

15. Albert Hofmann, speech at the International Symposium on LSD, Basel, 2006. As cited in "Bicycle Day & Albert Hofmann: Celebrating LSD and Modern Day Psychedelics," *Microdose* (April 2023): online.

the direct supervision of professionals, and as part of a broader psycho-therapy treatment. Given that psychedelics are very safe substances at a physiological level, but have psychological risks, especially in certain people, they are usually only administered to patients who have already tried other treatments without success, who have undergone a psycho-logical screening process to rule out latent illnesses (such as psychotic disorders or bipolarity), and who undergo psychological preparation sessions prior to the psychedelic experience, always following safety protocols.[16]

After the experience, in which the person has remained with their eyes closed, with headphones on and a selected music playlist, and in the company and supervision of a team of professionals, an integration process is carried out that is a crucial step to work with all the material that emerged during the psychedelic experience.

What is important about this treatment model is that, unlike cur-rent treatments with antidepressants or anxiolytics, where the drug is taken daily, masking the symptoms, in psychedelic-assisted psychother-apy the substance is only administered in one or two sessions through-out the entire treatment, the aim being to induce a transformative experience in those sessions, the therapeutic results of which last long after the therapy is finished. That is to say, the psychedelic would only act as a catalyst, facilitating that transformative and lasting experience, favoring access to the root of the problem and allowing therapist and patient to work on it. A psychotherapeutic process that normally might take months or even years happens in a few sessions.

And, indeed, most of this research is concluding that psychedelics, administered in a context of psychotherapy under direct professional supervision and in a controlled environment, are capable of catalyzing such transformative experiences, associated with long-lasting therapeu-tic results (that could last for years), quickly, safely (if done in well pre-pared patients), and effectively. In many cases, this therapy achieves the

---

16. M. W. Johnson, W. A. Richards, and R. R. Griffiths, "Human Hallucinogen Research: Guidelines for Safety," *Journal of Psychopharmacology* 22, no. 6 (August 2008): 603–20.

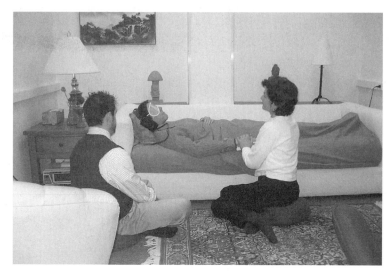

Psilocybin-assisted psychotherapy session at Johns Hopkins University.
There are usually two therapists (female and male) to provide support
throughout the session. Photo by Matthew W. Johnson,
via the Research Outreach website.

partial or complete remission of some mental disorders such as depression, anxiety, post-traumatic stress disorder, and addictions in patients who have not managed to improve with conventional therapies.

These types of disorders, nowadays, usually require very extensive, expensive conventional therapeutic processes and long-term pharmacological treatments, sometimes with unwanted side effects. Following these control and supervision guidelines, the safety, effectiveness, and durability rates that are being achieved in psychedelic research are above the best current conventional treatments, with fewer side effects and in much less time. Nevertheless, more research is still required to consolidate these results with psychedelics, given that at the moment most studies are carried out with very small groups of patients, in very specific conditions, and, given the intensity of the psychedelic experience, it is difficult to blind participants about whether they received the psychedelic or the placebo, making it very difficult to rule out the effects of expectancy.

To discuss and make all this research visible, a growing number of conferences, conventions, and annual scientific congresses are organized

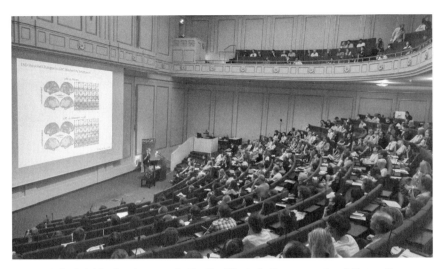

INSIGHT 2021 Conference, in Berlin. Photo is the property of the author.
(See also color plate 5.)

to serve as a space for meeting and disseminating the latest advances in this field, such as Psychedelic Science, Breaking Convention, ICPR, Horizons, World Ayahuasca Conference, Beyond Psychedelics, INSIGHT, and many others.

As proof of the rapid change in attitude that regulatory agencies such as the EMA or the FDA have had regarding psychedelic drugs, thanks to this scientific development, aided by better access to information and the experience of previous regulatory processes (such as medical cannabis), the stigmas surrounding research with psychedelics are disappearing, making the original impediments—legal, economic, technical and social—turn into advantages. As an example, the fact that the FDA (Food and Drug Administration) is approving the breakthrough therapy designation for many of these trials based on their safety and efficacy, which is accelerating their development and medical authorization. Now this whole field is being greatly boosted with milestones that would be unimaginable just five years ago:

- Esketamine (enantiomer of ketamine), from Janssen Pharmaceuticals, was the first compound to be authorized for psychedelic therapy, in 2019 by the FDA and the EMA, for the treatment of treatment-resistant depression, and is marketed for medical use under the name Spravato in the form of a nasal spray in the United States, Europe, and many other countries. Likewise, racemic ketamine (the regular ketamine used in anesthesia for more than fifty years, containing a mixture of both esketamine and arketamine) has long been used in mental health treatments as an off-label treatment at doctors' discretion.

- Psilocybin, from the Compass Pathways pharmaceutical company, is already in phase 3[17] clinical trials for the treatment of major depression and could be authorized for controlled medical use in the next two years.

- The study of psilocybin for the treatment of smoking has just received a major grant from the National Institute on Drug Abuse (NIDA) in the United States to continue evaluating its efficacy and safety in this addictive disorder.

- MDMA, hand in hand with the NGO MAPS (now Lykos Therapeutics), concluded phase 3 clinical trials for treating PTSD in 2023 and an NDA (New Drug Application) was presented to the FDA in early 2024 that was deemed insufficient in August 2024, so a new phase 3 trial is being planned that will probably lead to its authorization for controlled medical use in the next few years.

- And there are many other psychedelic substances (ibogaine, DMT, ayahuasca, LSD, 5-MeO-DMT, psilocybin, and MDMA) currently being investigated or considered for many other therapeutic conditions (addictions, social anxiety, anorexia, tinnitus, phobias, anxiety, obsessive-compulsive disorder, dementia, Alzheimer's, stuttering, long COVID, palliative care, and chronic pain, among others) and that are in different states and phases of development and authorization, so it seems that this revolution in the research and medical use of psychedelics has only just begun.

- In July 2023 the TGA from Australia authorized the use of both MDMA and psilocybin in treating PTSD and depression respectively, keeping both drugs as unapproved therapeutic goods with tight restrictions on their indications, who can prescribe them (approved

---

17. Clinical trials prior to the approval of a new drug are divided into phases 1, 2, and 3.

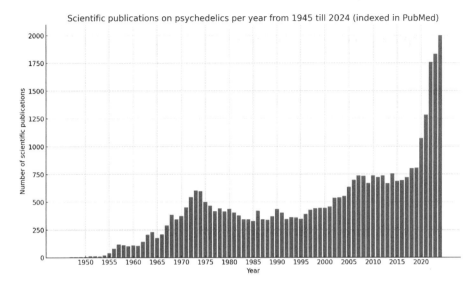

Number of scientific publications on psychedelics in PubMed (on the y-axis) per year (on the x-axis), clearly showing that the "psychedelic renaissance" has already surpassed the research of the 1960s and 1970s. Graph made by the author with data from PubMed.

psychiatrists only), and the conditions under which they can be used, requiring the approval and oversight of an ethics committee.

To give an idea of the magnitude of this scientific phenomenon, more than half of all scientific research on psychedelics ever published has come in the last decade, with those publications carried out in the United Kingdom, United States, Switzerland, Spain, and Brazil having the greatest impact so far.[18]

The popular magazine *Science* included trials in MDMA-assisted psychotherapy for the treatment of post-traumatic stress in its list of the ten greatest advances in science in 2021,[19] while many universities and research institutions have already gone beyond their psychedelic research programs

18. Aviad Hadar et al., "The Psychedelic Renaissance in Clinical Research: A Bibliometric Analysis of Three Decades of Human Studies with Classical Psychedelics," *Journal of Psychoactive Drugs* 55 no. 9 (January 2022): 1–10.
19. Kelly Servick, "2021 Breakthrough of the Year - A Psychedelic PTSD Remedy," *Science* (December 2021): online.

and have founded specialized centers. Some examples are the Johns Hopkins University Center for Psychedelic and Consciousness Research; the Imperial College London's Centre for Psychedelic Research; the University of California, Berkeley Center for the Science of Psychedelics; Neuroscape at the University of California, San Francisco; the Center for Psychedelic Research & Therapy at Dell Medical School (part of the UT Austin Medical Center); the Massachusetts General Hospital Center for the Neuroscience of Psychedelics; the NYU Langone Health Center for Psychedelic Medicine; the Center for Psychedelic Psychotherapy and Trauma Research at the Icahn School of Medicine at Mount Sinai; the Michigan Psychedelic Center at the University of Michigan; the Center for Psychedelic Research at the University of Zurich; and more.

In short, we are currently in a golden era for research with psychedelics, a moment that the first article on the subject in a mainstream publication of relevance in 2010 called a "Psychedelic Renaissance,"[20] baptizing this revolution in research and giving rise to what we are seeing today in the field of research, but also to what is being experienced

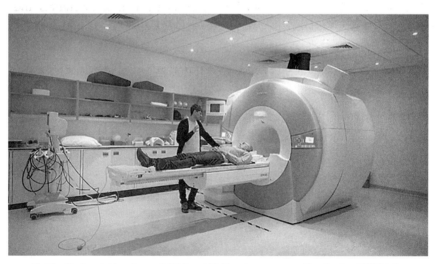

Robin Carhart-Harris and Michael Pollan in conversation in the fMRI lab, Imperial Center for Psychedelic Research. Photo by Thomas Angus, Imperial College London.

---

20. Steven Kotler, "The New Psychedelic Renaissance," *Playboy* (April 2010): 51–52.

in other fields. As was the case in the 1960s and 1970s, this originally scientific movement is already becoming social, cultural, political, and industrial, permeating very diverse fields and promoting new business, technological, cultural, informative, and legal initiatives, which implies greater social interest and visibility but, at the same time, could become a threat if the sociocultural phenomena of the past were to occur again.

SOCIAL AND CULTURAL CONTEXTS

Since approximately 2015, references to psychedelics in the press, books, magazines, and documentaries have multiplied. Reputable popularizers, such as Michael Pollan, the prestigious writer and journalist, began to publish[21] on the subject in all kinds of mass media, and people unfamiliar with the field of psychedelics or other illegal substances became interested.

For years, the traditional, ceremonial, and therapeutic use of psychedelics with strong cultural roots outside the West, such as ayahuasca, peyote, iboga, and many others, had already been spreading throughout the world, allowing those interested to come into contact with these substances and their traditional medicinal uses and further disseminate its associated values and cultural elements; but in recent years they have become more visible and accessible and have had a greater sociocultural impact outside the field of anthropological research, for example as a spiritual and self-development tool.

The growing interest of society in the field of psychedelics is stimulating the appearance of more and more outreach initiatives in this field: new media like *Psychedelic Times*; magazines like *Double Blind Mag*; resources following the psychedelic revival such as *Psychedelics Alpha*; documentaries like *Have a Good Trip, How to Change Your Mind, DOSED, or Nine Perfect Strangers*; bestsellers like *How to Change Your Mind* (the basis for the 2022 documentary);[22] and podcasts like *Psychedelics Today*.[23]

---

21. Michael Pollan, "The Trip Treatment," *The New Yorker* (February 1, 2015): online.
22. Michael Pollen, *How to Change Your Mind: What the New Science of Psychedelics Teaches Us about Consciousness, Dying, Addiction, Depression, and Transcendence* (New York: Penguin, 2019).
23. The titles of many of these resources are available in the Psychedelic Resources section of this book.

Other big mainstream podcasts often mention this topic, like *The Joe Rogan Experience* or *The Huberman Lab*. Also new apps have emerged like Mindleap Health and Maya, and thousands of news articles are being published on the subject by the mainstream media, like *The New York Times*, CNN, the BBC, and *The Washington Post*. Likewise, more and more organizations and universities are creating courses, centers, and specific groups for training and working with psychedelics.

In this context, "psychedelic societies"[24] are flourishing in most cities in the world,[25] allowing anyone with an interest in these substances to join, learn, and contribute to this renaissance. All of this, together with the decentralized dissemination of information that the internet and its forums allow, has given the general population access to much firsthand information on these substances. Thanks to resources such as PsychonautWiki, TripSit, Erowid, Bluelight, Drugs-Forum, Drogopedia, or Energy Control, anyone outside the academic field can access scientific information on substances and risk reduction techniques, which would have been very difficult to find years ago.

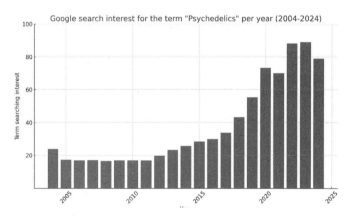

Increase in Google searches for "psychedelics" between 2004 and 2024. Graph created by the author. (See also color plate 9.)

---

24. Association model that has sprouted in various cities around the world to bring together people with an interest in learning, disseminating, doing activism and social relations for a common interest.

25. A directory of these societies is available in the Psychedelic Resources section of this book.

Similar to what happened with cannabis twenty-five years ago, we are now again witnessing a number of popular legal initiatives that are facilitating the therapeutic use and decriminalizing the possession and use of psychedelics in various U.S. cities and states (such as Oregon, Colorado, Massachusetts, and California). In certain aspects, psychedelics seem to be following a similar evolution to that of therapeutic cannabis in its day, although given its characteristics, quite different access models and therapeutic objectives are being pursued. In the case of psychedelics, their decriminalization is running in parallel with their pharmaceutical and industrial development, and the possibility of their non-medical or even recreational use is not always viewed favorably by the scientific community, since these are extremely powerful substances with potentially bigger risks if used without proper professional control, and their non-clinical use could itself become a risk factor that could lead to repeating the events of the 1960s.

For example, in late 2020, Oregon voted and passed two legislative initiatives (109 and 110) aimed at decriminalizing illegal drugs and legalizing the therapeutic administration of psilocybin, becoming the first region in the world to expressly legalize the therapeutic administration of a psychedelic through a state program. Also, after authorizing the use of psilocybin in terminal patients, Canada recently authorized the administration of psilocybin by doctors to patients with any treatment-resistant condition in specific circumstances, although it is still facing many obstacles to implementing this new legislation, and an increasing number of dispensaries are now offering psilocybin mushrooms. But the most ambitious step was taken by Australia in July 2023 when the TGA authorized the use of both MDMA and psilocybin in PTSD and depression respectively, keeping both drugs as unapproved therapeutic goods, under tight restrictions on their indications, who can prescribe them (approved psychiatrists only), and the conditions under which they can be used, requiring the approval and oversight of an ethics committee.

The internet and various media outlets are also creating and giving visibility to some personalities of this movement. Without going any further, in recent years a list of the current 100 most influential living people of the psychedelic renaissance was published, mainly focused on the United States, but including some international names as well, yet not including most of those who were active at the beginning of the research (some people already mentioned earlier in this chapter). Some of the people this list considers most influential today are: activist-scientists who started the movement and continue to have a huge impact like Rick Doblin (founder of MAPS), David Nichols (scientist and founder of the Heffter Research Institute), Amanda Feilding (founder of the Beckley Foundation), Stanislav Grof (developer of transpersonal psychology), James Fadiman (Institute of Transpersonal Psychology and Sofia University), or the mycologist Paul Stamets (Fungi Perfecti); great communication figures and supporters of relevance such as Tim Ferriss (*The Tim Ferriss Show*), Joe Rogan (*The Joe Rogan Experience*, UFC), Sam Harris (*Making Sense* Podcast), and Jordan B. Peterson; writers and journalists like Michael Pollan, Hamilton Morris (Vice); artists like Alex Grey; famous athletes like Mike Tyson and Lamar Odom; philanthropists, investors, businessmen, billionaires, and even politicians like former presidential candidate Andrew Yang. It also mentions some personalities from the world of clinical psychedelic science such as Robin Carhart-Harris (former Imperial College London and current University of California, San Francisco), Rick Strassman (University of New Mexico), David Nutt (Imperial College London), Rosalind Watts (Imperial College London), Matthew Johnson (Johns Hopkins University), Roland Griffiths (Johns Hopkins University), and Ben Sessa (Awakn), leaving in the inkwell a large number of very important people at the scientific level who are less visible nowadays in mainstream media.

Also, various celebrities of film, music, television, and sports—not mentioned in the previous list—have "come out of the psychedelic closet" recounting their therapeutic psychedelic experiences, as is the case of Sting, Seth Rogen, Miley Cyrus, Will Smith, Paul McCartney, Paul Simon, Megan Fox, Gwyneth Paltrow, Ben Lee, Daniel Carcillo, and Kristen Bell.

Before the pandemic, and even more after, the popularity of psychedelic-themed festivals such as Burning Man, BOOM, Psy-Fi or O.Z.O.R.A Festival is at an all-time high, as is the demand for risk reduction and care services for difficult psychedelic trips (known as "emergency trip-sitting services") carried out by organizations that emerged within these festivals, such as Kosmicare in Portugal or the Zendo Project in the United States, and new services such as remote assistance in difficult trips from the Fireside Project or TripSit, together with other essential risk reduction tools, such as information and drug analysis, provided by organizations such as Energy Control, Unity, Échele Cabeza, Dance Safe, and Safe'n Sound.

This renaissance also has its own "International Celebration Day," a cause for all kinds of meetings and celebrations. April 19, known worldwide as Bicycle Day, commemorates Albert Hofmann's bicycle ride in Basel, Switzerland, on April 19, 1943, from his laboratory to his home, where he began to feel "strange" after having intentionally ingested, for the first time in history, a dose of LSD.

Some surveys such as the Global Drug Survey have already shown from 2020 an increase in the number of people who say they are using psychedelics recreationally or to treat different mental health disorders at home, which logically generates discomfort in some circles that fear that consumption of these substances without adequate knowledge and control can cause problems. A recent survey on psychedelics by the UC Berkeley Center for the Science of Psychedelics (BCSP) found that more than six in ten (61 percent) of American registered voters support legalizing regulated therapeutic access to psychedelics, including 35 percent who report "strong" support. Over half of voters polled (56 percent) support obtaining FDA approval for psychedelics by prescription. Forty-seven percent of voters have heard something about psychedelics recently and over half (51 percent) reported a "first-degree" connection to psychedelic use—that either they or someone close to them has used a psychedelic. In addition, more than three-quarters of voters (78 percent) support making it easier for researchers to study psychedelic substances. Almost half (49 percent) support removing criminal penalties for personal use and possession, with support for spiritual and religious use polling at just over four out of ten voters (44 percent).[26]

---

26. "UC Berkeley Center for the Science of Psychedelics Unveils Results of the First-Ever Berkeley Psychedelics Survey" (July 2023), via the UC Berkeley Center for the Science of Psychedelics website.

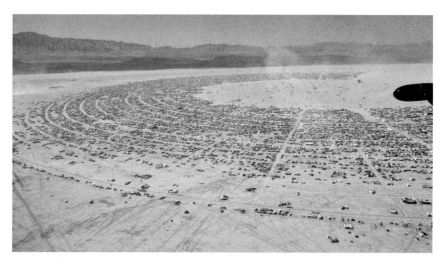

Aerial view of the Burning Man festival, in Black Rock, Nevada.
Photo by Steve Jurvetson.

At the moment, it is difficult to know the specific social impact of the popularization of psychonautical culture and "DIY" psychedelic-assisted psychotherapy. A recent study found that 3.1 percent of Americans aged eighteen and older (approximately 8 million people) used psilocybin in 2023.[27] We know it is a subject that is already being discussed with greater interest in forums and raising more questions, as there is greater and greater ease for disseminating and accessing information on the domestic cultivation of mushrooms or simple DMT extraction techniques, with the possibility to easily find companies that facilitate home production for self-consumption. Furthermore, in recent years, this revolution also coincided with an increase in the availability and purity of psychedelics, such as LSD, MDMA, and DMT, on the unregulated market, as well as the appearance of new synthetic psychedelic substances that are not controlled yet in many countries and are very affordable, such as 1P-LSD and 4-AcO-DMT,[28] which may further facilitate accessibility to psychedelics.

27. Beau Kilmer, Michelle Priest, Rajeev Ramchand, Rhianna C. Rogers, Ben Senator, and Keytin Palmer, "Considering Alternatives to Psychedelic Drug Prohibition," RAND Corporation Research Report (June 2024): online.
28. European Monitoring Centre for Drugs and Drug Addiction, "European Drug Report 2021: Trends and Developments" (September 2021): online.

But what does seem clear is that this rapid popularization in the West, where, unlike other cultures, there is still no good social understanding of the handling of psychedelic substances, their use outside controlled clinical settings could lead us to repeat the unfortunate events from the 1960s. We must not forget that "classic" psychedelics, despite being pharmacologically safe substances at the physiological level, can pose great risks at the psychological level—if they are administered without prior screenings that can rule out a propensity for psychosis or bipolarity, without prior preparation, or in a context without adequate control by professionals, or if no subsequent integration of the experience is provided.

Our modern societies are not yet used to handling these substances, just as there are other societies that may be used to them, but may not be used to, let's say, alcohol. Whenever a new psychoactive substance enters a society that is unaware of it, the risk potential is much greater than when it is already part of that culture and its handling is known by the majority of the population.

THE RISE OF A NEW INDUSTRY

The relationship of psychedelic substances with Silicon Valley and with the great centers of technological innovation is nothing new, and in this sense, another event that contributed to resurrecting these substances in the field of technological innovation was the report in which Steve Jobs, the most important technological entrepreneur in history and creator of the most valued company, Apple, declared:

Taking LSD was a profound experience, one of the most important things in my life. LSD shows you that there is another side to the coin, and you can't remember it when it wears off, but you know it. It reinforced my sense of what was important—creating great things instead of making money, putting things back into the stream of history and of human consciousness as much as I could.[29]

29. Walter Isaacson, *Steve Jobs* (New York: Simon & Schuster, 2011); see page 46.

When Apple started working for the U.S. government in the 1980s, Steve Jobs had to be investigated by the Department of Defense and underwent a background check to obtain a top-secret security clearance (recently declassified and published) in which he also defended the positive contribution of psychedelics to his life.

Along these same lines, at the end of 2021, Elon Musk, CEO of Space X, Tesla, and the richest man in the world, declared at an event:

> I think, generally, people should be open to psychedelics. A lot of people making laws are kind of from a different era, so I think, as the new generation gets into political power, we'll see a greater receptivity to the benefits of psychedelics.[30]

Years later, in 2024, Musk also declared in an interview he was using prescribed ketamine treatments to manage his mental health, particularly to handle depression, by using a small amount of ketamine approximately once every other week as part of his treatment plan. These statements by the most famous entrepreneurs of our time join those already made by investor, writer, and polymath Tim Ferriss to CNN Money a few years ago, in which he said that the billionaires he knows "almost without exception, use hallucinogens on a regular basis, trying to be very disruptive and look at the problems of the world . . . and ask completely new questions."

The use of psychedelic substances aimed at improving creativity, productivity, and work in general is also currently trending—changing the stereotype of the user from "hippie" to "yuppie." An exponent of this trend is the emergence of some practices that do not seek transformative experiences, but rather integrate the potential of psychedelics with the workplace, as is the case of microdosing, an apparently popular practice in Silicon Valley, startups, and other innovation ecosystems, which consists of taking small, minimal, sub-perceptual doses[31]

---

30. Elon Musk, "People Should Be Open to Psychedelics," CodeCon 2021, September 2021.
31. Below the minimum detectable amount.

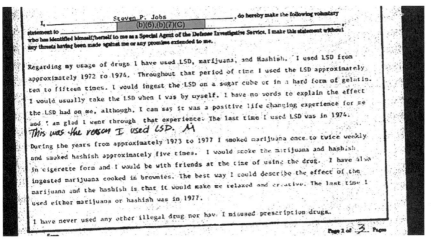

Steve Jobs declared: "I used LSD from approximately 1972 to 1974. Throughout that period of time I used the LSD approximately ten to fifteen times. I would ingest the LSD in a sugar cube or in a hard form of gelatin. I would usually take the LSD when I was by myself. I have no words to explain the effect the LSD had on me, although, I can say that it was a positive life-changing experience for me and I am glad that I went through that experience." Image from "Steve Jobs' Pentagon File: Blackmail Fears, Youthful Arrest and LSD Cubes," 2012, via WIRED online.

of psychedelics on a regular basis to go to work or perform creative activities, with some people reporting they improve productivity, mood, habits, and relationships.[32] Despite the fact that, according to the scarce research published so far, it is still not clear if the microdoses have positive pharmacological effects exceeding the placebo effect, it is a practice the media has reported as very common (there has even been a high-level dismissal related to it), and it already has some resources dedicated exclusively to it as The Third Wave, although it has very little evidence so far and there are still many unknowns about its real effectiveness compared to placebos.[33] Microdosing is not only being used and studied for work-related goals, it's also being widely used as a therapeutic tool,

32. Aylet Waldman, *A Really Good Day: How Microdosing Made a Mega Difference in My Mood, My Marriage, and My Life* (Anchor, 2017).
33. Balázs Szigeti et al., "Self-Blinding Citizen Science to Explore Psychedelic Microdosing," *eLife* 10 (March 2021): e62878.

but, contrary to the psychedelic-assisted psychotherapies with mega-doses, these microdoses lack scientific evidence of efficacy yet.

This is why there is often talk of a paradoxical evolution of the stereotype of the person who consumes psychedelics, from the image of the hippie of the 1960s, associated with spiritual, ecological, and human development, to the yuppie of today, with a professional drive to improve creativity and productivity, using psychedelics to work more and not to work less, while others use psychedelics as a way to keep sanity and cope with a crazy world.

But there is not only an interest in its use associated with work and creativity—psychedelics themselves represent the emergence of a new industry. Although the therapeutic model of psychedelic-assisted psychotherapy may seem less exploitable from a commercial perspective compared to other models in the traditional pharmaceutical industry, due to the fact that the psychedelic substance is only administered a couple of times throughout the treatment (as opposed to the daily use of common treatments with antidepressants or anxiolytics), and with fewer opportunities for patenting (because most classic psychedelics are natural, or were synthetized a long time ago and are currently off-patent), this has not prevented the emergence of innovative startups and new pharmaceutical companies in recent years (such as Compass Pathways, MindMed, Cybin, Atai, Numinus, Havn Life, Beckley Psytech, or Mydecine Innovations). These, in addition to supporting clinical research in the field, are even achieving great results on Wall Street and other exchanges, obtaining billions of dollars in financing, which is clear evidence of the interest in this subject and its future development, which some analysts predict will exceed ten thousand million dollars in the next few years.

However, more clinical research is still needed, together with better regulation and financing of these treatments, as well as deepening the debates on the future coexistence of regulated and medicalized commercial models with the ancestral cultural practices of the use of psychedelics that some societies still maintain. The Western pharmaceutical development of these substances is not without some controversy or ethical debates, as was clearly seen in many forums as well as at the closing event of Psychedelic Science 2023 in Denver, Colorado, where some activists interrupted the closing ceremony by Rick Doblin to voice their concerns regarding the Western medical development of what they consider their traditional medicines. And some of these concerns were seen again during various milestones by the psychedelic pharmaceutical industry and the regulatory developments in different cities and states.

"Psychedelic tourism" and traditional healing centers managed by small initiatives of traditional use, like the Takiwasi Center or the Temple of the Way of Light (both in Peru), or large companies, such as Beckley Retreats, Spinoza, and the Synthesis and Essence Institutes, and groups that offer retreats with ayahuasca and other psychedelic compounds or the possibility of participating in ceremonies are now very accessible in many places. Their services are demanded by many people with various profiles, from people with simple curiosity, to those seeking self-exploration, spirituality, and therapy, and even celebrities, billionaires, and CEOs. Modern clinics that already work with ketamine legally have also been established in Western countries and offer their services in a highly professional manner, as is the case with Field Trip Health, Numinus, and Infuse RVa, while awaiting authorization for medical use of other psychedelic substances to add those to the therapeutic toolbox. Also, a new trend is offering at-home ketamine sessions, with virtual guiding; this format, offered by companies like Nue Life, Mindbloom, Better U Care, and Wondermed, is more convenient but also might be more risky due to the lack of in-person professional supervision.

In short, this new industry and its various ramifications are trending and seem to have a promising future, especially in the clinical and pharmaceutical fields, but also in the sociocultural field. Although it will take some time to see all the aspects and enduring developments of this psychedelic renaissance, it is very likely that many innovations and developments will continue to appear in all these areas in the coming years.

5

How Psychedelics Work

It is not the purpose of this book to delve much into the mechanisms of action of psychedelics, a very technical subject widely addressed in other books. It would also require us to explain, in much greater depth, the functioning of the brain. Instead, I will give a global and simplified idea of the effects and mechanisms that underlie an altered state of consciousness induced by psychedelic substances. This will make it easier to fully understand the psychotherapeutic potential of these substances and how they can change us—temporarily or lastingly.

Although we still cannot fully detail all the mechanisms of action of these compounds in the human brain, new research is published almost every month that improves our understanding of the brain under the influence of psychedelics and their potential clinical applications, so the evolution in this field is the order of the day.

MECHANISMS AT THE NEURORECEPTOR LEVEL

As we have seen before, psychedelic compounds (also known as hallucinogens or entheogens) are a specific group of psychoactive substances that come from various chemical families, both of natural origin (present in plants, fungi, and even animals), semi-synthetic (small modifications from the natural molecule), and totally synthetic. They have the capacity to induce altered states of consciousness through, fundamentally, the activation of neuronal serotonin receptors (more specifically, those of the 5-HT2a class).

From left to right: serotonin, psilocybin, DMT, and LSD. Molecules with psychedelic effects resemble serotonin, and therefore fit into its neuroreceptors, particularly the 5-HT2a receptor.

Although some psychedelic substances may be atypical (such as ketamine or MDMA) and produce these effects by different routes with different quality, for the purpose of explaining their brain mechanisms I will stick to the classic psychedelics (psilocybin, LSD, and DMT), which share their direct action on this neuroreceptor of the serotonin system precisely because they resemble this neurotransmitter in some areas and "fit" into its "locks."

We know the importance of the 5-HT2a receptor because numerous studies carried out in animals and humans[1] show that the substances with the greatest affinity for the 5-HT2a receptor are the ones that produce the greatest psychedelic effect, while antagonistic substances (blockers) of this receptor (such as ketanserin) can eliminate the psychedelic effect of any of these drugs.

These 5-HT2a receptors are mostly in the cerebral cortex, the outer layer of the brain (which humans have disproportionally larger than any other animal). This layer is responsible for high-level cognitive functions, such as analytical, abstract, and associative thinking, among others. The proportion of the number of 5-HT2a receptors activated by a psychedelic in the cortex is directly correlated to the intensity of the psychedelic experience in a person. When approximately more than sixty percent of these receptors are activated is when

---

1. Katrin H. Preller et al., "Changes in Global and Thalamic Brain Connectivity in LSD-Induced Altered States of Consciousness are Attributable to the 5-HT2A Receptor," *eLife* 7 (October 2018): e35082.

the psychedelic effects with the most therapeutic interest begin to occur, such as "ego dissolution," and "mystical experiences."[2] In short, the more 5-HT2a receptors are activated in the cerebral cortex, the greater the intensity of psychedelic effects that will be produced; and for most of the therapeutic effects to be produced, a threshold has to be exceeded, which will trigger transient but profound changes in brain connectivity.

MECHANISMS AT THE BRAIN LEVEL

Before, I mentioned that one of the factors that is making this psychedelic renaissance possible is a better understanding of their mechanisms of action, thanks, among other things, to modern neuroimaging techniques such as PET or fMRI.

When scientists began to look at the brain under the influence of psychedelics like psilocybin or LSD, they expected to find that they activated different cortical regions. Instead, they found that they produced a decrease in activity in certain brain regions, specifically in a network known as the default mode network (DMN) and that this decrease in activity affected the way the rest of the brain worked. They also noticed that this was highly correlated with the psychedelic effects perceived by the individual (ego dissolution, connection, synesthesia). For this reason, they hypothesized that the DMN was the main area in the brain where psychedelics exerted their action. Based on these observations, work began on a theory explaining why these effects occur when reducing DMN activity and what this tells us about brain function. One of the most updated and complete theories on these effects is the unified model REBUS and the anarchic brain[3] (relaxed beliefs under psychedelics), built upon a revised version of the

---

2. A mystical experience is a very personal introspective experience in which some kind of universal unity or transcendence of time and space is described.

3. R. L. Carhart-Harris and K. J. Friston, "REBUS and the Anarchic Brain: Toward a Unified Model of the Brain Psychedelics," *Pharmacological Reviews* 71, no. 3 (July 2019): 316–44.

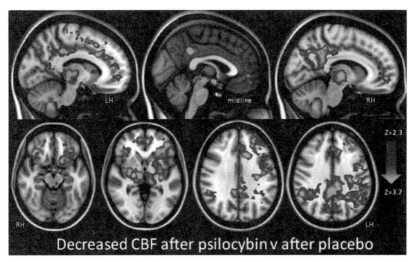

Decreased CBF after psilocybin v after placebo

Temporary decrease in blood flow and activation in certain brain regions after psilocybin. Regions shown are those that had a significant decrease when exposed to psilocybin compared to placebo. Image from Carhart-Harris et al., "Neural Correlates of the Psychedelic State as Determined by fMRI Studies with Psilocybin," *Proceedings of the National Academy of Sciences* 109, no. 6 (January 2012): 2138–43. Used with permission from Carhart-Harris. (See also color plate 3.)

entropic brain theory[4] by Robin Carhart-Harris,[5] and the free energy principle[6] by Karl Friston. I will not delve into them, but they will be the basis on which I will support a very simplified explanation of the mechanisms of action of these substances at the brain level.

HOW DOES THE BRAIN WORK?
HIERARCHICAL PREDICTIVE CODING

Our brain works like a machine to reduce the uncertainty of the world around us. It does this not only by continuously interpreting

---

4. Robin L. Carhart-Harris et al., "The Entropic Brain: A Theory of Conscious States Informed by Neuroimaging Research with Psychedelic Drugs," *Frontiers in Human Neuroscience* 8 (February 2014): 20.

5. Robin L. Carhart-Harris, "The Entropic Brain—Revisited," *Neuropharmacology* 142 (November 2018): 167–78.

6. Karl Friston, "The free-energy principle: A unified brain theory?" *Nature Reviews Neuroscience* 11, no. 2 (February 2010): 127–38.

our changing environment, in order to give quick responses that guarantee our survival, but also by constantly making predictions of the world around us based on models[7] and beliefs created by past experience—always using as little sensory information as possible—in order to save energy and time. Then, it compares those predictions with the reality that comes through the senses and see if they match.

Thus, it can build complex stories about the world that surrounds us with little sensory information, less consumption of resources, and saving time, by generating predictions in advance, which increases our probability of survival and adaptation. This is called predictive coding.

The brain improves in this task of prediction as it becomes an adult and develops and tests its models better against reality, learning the world around it and elevating these "confirmed" models in the hierarchy of brain processes. The problem is, in exchange for this efficiency, our thinking becomes "rigid" by creating models of fixed predictions (automated and efficient) based on past experiences that are very powerful, but which, in turn, limit us and influence our experience of the present outside reality.

These models and beliefs are like the colored lenses through which we see the world. There comes a time when these models that we build become so powerful that they also control the information (external and internal) that reaches them: they filter it out and prevent us from "seeing" some things, so we begin to perceive a reality that is highly influenced by our beliefs and experiences, one that can be very far from objective reality. If our predictive models become maladaptive and show us a world that is too negative or difficult, it can sometimes make it hard to live a healthy, fulfilling, and happy life.

In other words, when we are born, we do not have models, beliefs, or patterns about how the world works around us, but, since we need them to be able to adapt to the environment and survive, our brains begin to develop and structure themselves based on the information coming in

---

7. A model is a simplified version of something. The brain needs models to work efficiently and effectively, and not be overwhelmed by all the sensory input it continually receives.

during that stage. As this task is slow and very costly energetically, if we remained in this state of experimentation and constant observation, we would not survive long, so the brain learns and automates what it is able to verify, that is, it creates models with what it sees, feels, and experiences, and starts to make predictions based on those models. At first, these predictions fail a lot, but they improve with the accumulation of experience and end up being established as our models of the world.

All this psychological process is also neurological and morphological, and, as it progresses, our brain is "carved," creating structures and hierarchies. Neural networks with superior functions emerge that impose their operation and their learned models (their world view) on networks with more basic functions, such as sensory ones, which are limited to receiving information. And even though this information is more objective, it is too abundant to continuously process all of it in real time. The function of these networks of superior hierarchy and their models is very important, since without them we could not go from contemplating the world with fascination as a child to anticipating it and acting on it as an adult.

When we reach adulthood, our brain is a structure of hierarchical networks, both morphologically and functionally. This means that we have high-ranking neural networks that control, modulate, or limit the action of other hierarchically "inferior" neural networks, filtering their information and deciding what is relevant and what is not, anticipating what might happen, planning, and acting accordingly. We call this hierarchical predictive coding.

For example, at the base of this hierarchy are the sensory circuits that bring us information from the senses, from the outside world, with hardly any processing; and at the top would be networks such as the default mode network, which is considered the seat of the ego, and which is activated when we are not doing any external tasks and we wander through our minds, absorbed in our plans, memories, or concerns.

Many optical illusions are based on deceiving these models and their predictions, such as the classic hollow mask illusion where we are presented with a hollow mask, and because we ignore which side is facing us, our brain will interpret and predict, based on the models it has

Scan the QR code to see a video by the Royal Institution of the hollow mask illusion, showing us how we are conditioned by our learning to make predictions about reality, sometimes erroneously, instead of simply interpreting all the information that comes to us from the outside world, which would be overwhelming to do continuously.

established throughout our lives, that the mask is facing us when in fact it could be facing away and we could be looking at its hollow interior.

With the limited ambivalent sensory information the brain is receiving, it makes a prediction based on our years of experience identifying faces, which are always oriented toward us. So it interprets that the mask is facing us, confirming the validity of the sensory information that corresponds to this idea as opposed to the one that does not, filtering and discarding that conflicting information because it contradicts what we have been seeing for years. Furthermore, it is not able to change that prediction until the mask starts to rotate and, after a few tenths of a second of confusion, the sensory information contradicting our pre-established model becomes undeniable, and our brain finally "listens" to it and reformulates its prediction: what we were looking at was actually the concave side of this hollow mask.

In an infant state, before we have these top-hierarchy predictive models built and in place, this optical illusion doesn't work,[8] and we are able to see the mask as it really is: concave.

But it also doesn't work in a psychedelic state, or in other altered states of consciousness that can occur, for example, in schizophrenia. In these states, the hollow mask does not deceive the brain. The sensory information prevails over the pre-established high-level models and

---

8. Aki Tsuruhara et al., "The Hollow-Face Illusion in Infancy: Do Infants See a Screen Based Rotating Hollow Mask as Hollow?" *i-Perception* 2, no. 5 (July 2011): 418–27.

beliefs that would normally modulate and filter its activity (imposing its learned predictions against the reality that it receives through the senses), but that in these states are diminished or absent.

Formerly, it was thought that psychedelic substances opened our "doors of perception" by removing the filters through which we experience the reality that our senses perceive, but today we know that this concept, although it may be somewhat accurate, is much broader and more complex.

In essence, psychedelics temporarily dismantle this hierarchical pyramid structure in charge of filtering our senses and predicting the world, making the adult brain more like that of a child: open, perceptive, flexible, imaginative, creative, and fanciful, giving us a window of opportunity to change some things. Now we will see how they do it.

HOW DO PSYCHEDELICS AFFECT OUR BRAIN FUNCTION?

As we have mentioned before, when someone takes a psychedelic, the activation of the 5-HT2a neuroreceptors (mainly) of the cortical neurons of their brain reduces the activity of one of those high-ranking neural networks, known as the default mode network (DMN). This area of the brain is considered the seat of the ego or "I," and it normally controls, filters, and constrains other lower neural networks (such as the sensory neural networks responsible for collecting all the information from the outside world through the senses). This neural network is by default a great communication center of the brain and acts as an orchestra conductor or as a traffic guard, coordinating communication and traffic between different areas of the brain and deciding which messages rise to our consciousness and which do not, filtering a good part of the subconscious cognitive flow and suppressing messages from other more primitive or less hierarchical areas of the brain.

In the absence of the control exerted by the DMN, the normal neuronal activity of the brain is destabilized and the lower hierarchical level networks that were limited, filtered, or controlled by it become disorganized and lose their habitual, structured functioning patterns.

(a)   (b)

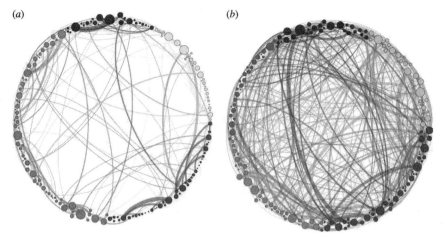

This representation shows the functional connectivity of different regions in a brain that has taken a placebo (a) versus a brain that has taken a dose of psilocybin (b). Image by G. Petri, P. Expert, F. Turkheimer, R. Carhart-Harris, D. Nutt, P. J. Hellyer, and F. Vaccarino. (See also color plate 10.)

The hierarchy of brain function ceases to be so pyramidal and becomes more horizontal. It dissolves, and various neural networks in the brain stop communicating with each other as independent clusters and begin to do so wholly, with all its regions, so that the functional connectivity of the brain as a whole increases and diversifies; it becomes interconnected. The brain begins to function in a more unified way, as we can see in the image above.[9]

The usual "highways" between specialized and compartmentalized areas of the brain disintegrate, while the brain, as a whole, integrates, becomes more globally interconnected and unified, more uniform and less specialized. It goes from using a few highways with few origins and destinations to using many, many smaller highways with many more origins and destinations, allowing regions of the brain that normally don't communicate with each other to do so, creating synesthesias,[10] hallucinations, novel connections, new ideas, and increasing creativity.

---

9. G. Petri et al., "Homological Scaffolds of Brain Functional Networks," *Journal of the Royal Society Interface* 11, no. 101 (December 2014): 20140873.

10. Synesthesia is the blending of senses: hearing a color, tasting a sound.

An analogy to understand this effect is to imagine neural signals as cars and neural pathways as highways. Under normal conditions, most traffic would circulate on highways to reach their usual destination faster, following the usual route and without looking at the landscape too much. But if we temporarily limit traffic on those usual highways with roadworks and make them more difficult to navigate, many cars will prefer to move on other secondary roads for some time. This will help rediscover new and old places (new restaurants, new landscapes, new paths), giving life to some towns that had been abandoned for years and, even though traffic may return to normal after a few hours, some of those secondary roads and their towns will have been brought back to life, with some drivers preferring to continue traveling through them. There will have been a lasting change in those models or routes because the knowledge obtained in this temporary experience will last for a long time, thanks to, among other things, an increase in neuroplasticity,[11] also induced by these drugs.

Another widely used analogy is to compare a psychedelic experience to what happens when you shake a snow globe. For a while that "snow" will be in a state of chaos, but it will settle again, although in a different way than it was at the beginning, which can be a great therapeutic opportunity.

By silencing the DMN, psychedelics act on our fundamental beliefs, allowing them to be influenced by lower hierarchies that are temporarily freed from the limitations imposed by the DMN. Sensory or memory areas (inferior to the DMN) are now able to send information without it being discarded by the "filter" of our beliefs and models, as infant brains do. In this process, the DMN becomes more malleable and, with this new information, can undergo lasting change, thereby effecting change to our models of the world, similar to updating the operating system of a computer. This puts the brain in what is known

---

11. Neuroplasticity is the flexibility of the brain's neural networks to adapt to changes, forming new connections (synapses) between neurons or modifying existing ones. Learning or memory are forms of neuroplasticity. Neuroplasticity is a capacity that decreases as the brain ages.

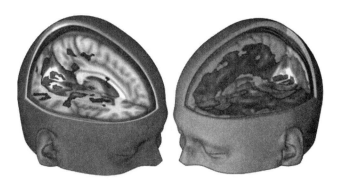

Imaging studies showed how LSD (right) increases connectivity between brain regions that do not communicate with each other under normal conditions (left). Image by Beckley/Imperial Research Program, from Carhart-Harris et al., "Neural Correlates of the LSD Experience Revealed by Multimodal Neuroimaging," *Proceedings of the National Academy of Sciences* 113, no. 17 (April 2016): 4853–58. Used with permission from Carhart-Harris. (See also color plate 11.)

as a pivotal mental state (like a bifurcation on the road, a crossroads), in which a change occurs that, depending on the conditions and the context of our mental state, may choose a path toward lasting change.

WHAT HAPPENS AT THE PSYCHOLOGICAL LEVEL?

Although at the cerebral level psychedelics "turn off" some regions and interconnect others, generating temporary chaos in the structures of the brain, the subjective phenomenology a person lives through during the psychedelic experience is enormously varied, creative, and subjective. It depends not only on the psychedelic that has been consumed and its dose, but, above all, on who the person is, their previous life experiences, mental and emotional state, present context, who is there too, and their intentions and expectations. In short, on their set and setting at the specific moment of ingestion. That is why no two psychedelic experiences are the same, and why the variables of person and context are so important when working with psychedelics, because the final experience and its results will depend on them.

The most characteristic psychological effects are significant changes in sensory perceptions, cognition, and consciousness.

In this informative chaos due to the absence of the DMN, the brain fluctuates between three options: allow the unfiltered passage of sensory information from neural networks hierarchically lower, also known as bottom-up (like looking at the hollow mask without interpreting that it is looking at us, that is, allowing uncertainty); impose its predictions based on its models (or top-down), risking being wrong, which would create predictive errors (hallucinations like seeing faces in the clouds) by trying to eliminate uncertainty at all costs; or simultaneously both processes, which supposes an overload of unfiltered information that the brain tries to make sense of through inaccurate predictions, returning to a primitive state of consciousness based more on "magical thinking."

Changes in sensory perceptions can manifest visually, with color enhancement, distortions in the shapes and movements of things, or colorful kaleidoscopic visions with closed eyes. Synesthesia (blending of the senses, like smelling colors or seeing sounds), increased tactile, thermal, or tingling sensations may appear. Hearing disturbances can lead to an increased appreciation of music and sounds. Also, there may be a noticeable increase in tactile, olfactory, or taste sensations. All of these symptoms can lead a person to laugh, achieve a state of wonder, confusion, or anxiety.

Cognitive alterations can be perceived as positive and pleasant or negative and difficult, and it is common for psychedelic experiences to include good stages and more difficult moments during the same session, which is why they are called "trips." It is common for biographical and personal content to emerge, as well as relationships with people who are significant to the subject or thoughts and concerns they may have at the time.

In general, the reduction of the ego or death of the ego (as it has been called) that occurs after the deactivation of the DMN softens or erases the limits of our body—it facilitates an experience of fusion with the environment, of unity, of connection with everything, of love. Consciousness expands beyond the usual constrictions. Sensory perception and mental states are greatly amplified, allowing information normally filtered by our models and beliefs of the world, located in the DMN, to rise into our consciousness. Not surprisingly, the term "psychedelic" derives from Latin roots *psyche* (mind) and *delos* (manifest), referring to its ability to "manifest the mind" or the underlying mental processes. Psychedelics make the unconscious conscious, make the invisible visible. If we were to imagine our mind as an iceberg with the tip being the conscious mind and the submerged part being the unconscious, the psychedelic would lower the water level so that a greater percentage of our unconscious mental processes become conscious.

Furthermore, when the ego dissolves, we stop being the center of our universe, we see things from another perspective, without preconceptions, and feelings of connection and deep universal love for everything can emerge, accompanied by well-being and joy. But feelings of anxiety or fear can also appear in the face of what can be perceived as a loss of identity, existence, or even sanity. The dissolution of the ego is perceived by itself like a big threat, like the end, and the person can feel it like dying.

This state of expanded consciousness is characterized by a feeling of being in the present and connection with what surrounds us or is within us at that moment, like a child who lives in the now, full of spontaneity. This contrasts with the adult ego state, which lives in the past or in the future, characterized by feelings of separation between us and what surrounds us, giving rise to fears, anxieties, remorse, repentance, defense, or haste. Many psychedelics can reduce the activity of the amygdala, the center of the brain related to fear and the fight-or-flight response, and thereby induce a positive bias in the perception of ourselves and our environment.

At high doses, the experience can rise to the level of what is known as a mystical experience, which is a deeply introspective and personal experience of ego and identity dissolution, including numinous feelings, a deeply positive emotional state, of internal unity, transcendence of time and space, ineffability and sensation of unity and interconnection with all things, along with oceanic-type feelings and universal love. This can be lived as experiences of death and rebirth, of surrender and acceptance, new purposes, senses, and meanings for life and the elements that make it up (for example, relationships, work, spirituality, or life goals).

All this subjective experience develops according to a specific narrative, which is what gives psychedelic experiences the name of "trips." That is why each trip is different, because it does not depend so much on the substance as on what is reaching our brain from the senses and from our own subconscious during the experience. Psychedelics temporarily open doors, but what passes through them depends greatly on the variables of person and context.

WHY DO WE HAVE 5-HT2A RECEPTORS AND PSYCHEDELIC EXPERIENCES?

There is much speculation about the original evolutionary role of the 5-HT2a neuroreceptor in particular and its possible function. We know that serotonin is released, for example, in response to stress, just as endorphins are released in response to pain. Therefore, it is logical to think that serotonin plays a role in stressful situations, and the activation of the 5-HT2a receptor, among others, does too.

Serotonin is closely related to our sensitivity to context, to the conditions in which we find ourselves, whether social (as numerous experiments with MDMA on humans and even octopuses have shown) or otherwise. This serotonin 5-HT2a system is usually active in our childhood development, but it is much less so when we reach maturity. So, it is speculated that it could be related to the establishment and progressive rigidity of our beliefs, models, and ways of thinking (and the neuroplasticity necessary to establish them), which become more effective and efficient but less flexible with age and experience. We become more efficient and fast in our predictions of the world, but we lose the ability to see and learn freely from what surrounds us, to think "outside of the box," and we filter the world through our lenses built from our experience, applying our bias to reality.

Therefore, psychedelics take our minds "outside of the box," making us extremely sensitive to our environment, be it our internal environment (set: thoughts, concerns, intentions, expectations, ideas, memories, subconscious) or the external physical and social context (setting: people, music, sounds, smells, images).

Likewise, the activation of the 5-HT2a receptor seems to increase brain plasticity, neuroplasticity, and even synaptogenesis and the growth of new branches in neurons, facilitating the acquisition or elimination of maladaptive learning (such as phobias), that is, changing and updating our models with information from our particular set and setting, again kind of like updating the operating system of a computer. Once the system enters this mode of learning and neuroplasticity, it becomes very sensitive to internal and environmental conditions. You could relearn from them like a child, you will become more likely to doubt your own previous beliefs-models, and you will be able to modify them in favor of new learning, being more open to change and adaptation.

One possibility that has been speculated is that the activation of these receptors acts as a reset button or as an update to our models that can be activated in extreme situations when we have to accelerate our adaptation to the environment, as would happen when we expose ourselves to any kind of stressful situation, like a near-death experience. In fact, we know that in animals, such experiences produce a marked increase in serotonin in the brain, as well as in DMT (a powerful psychedelic substance that is present in minute amounts in the brains of all mammals). This would be in line with some of the ideas laid out by Rick Strassman in his book *DMT: The Spirit Molecule*,[12] where he proposed its release in extreme situations, with an adaptive function—although this field is still quite speculative.

HOW CAN PSYCHEDELICS HELP WITH MENTAL HEALTH DISORDERS OR OTHER MALADAPTIVE CONDITIONS?

Many mental health disorders (such as depression, addictions, or OCD) are correlated to overactivity in the default mode network (DMN). In

---

12. Rick Strassman, *DMT: The Spirit Molecule: A Doctor's Revolutionary Research into the Biology of Near-Death and Mystical Experiences* (Rochester, VT: Inner Traditions/ Bear and Company, 2000).

other words, our high-hierarchy models of the world have become so rigid and maladaptive that they become pathological, excessively filtering and controlling the functioning of our brain, our behavior, our thinking, and our vision of the world. This disconnects us from the reality that surrounds us, pushing us to repeat patterns, constantly ruminate on thoughts in the first person, making it difficult for us to change and reinforcing our convictions and models, even if they are being harmful to us. They make us live more "inside" our brains and less in the outside world.

Changing those models, beliefs, or thought patterns is a very arduous and time-consuming task. However, during a psychedelic experience, these models and patterns break down, become more flexible, their hierarchy dissolves or becomes less pronounced, making it easier for abstract concepts to mix with sensory information and vice versa, and thus "updating" these models within a therapeutic context ideally.

Psychedelic substances act in the brain in such a way that they allow us to doubt those beliefs or high-ranking models, making them more flexible and reshaping them, updating them with external information coming from the senses or with internal information coming from our memory or from other neural networks of lower hierarchy than the DMN. This allows us to see new perspectives of things, remember things that we had forgotten, detect blind spots in our way of thinking that could be harming us and that are normally undetectable by us, filtered by the DMN and its models, or help us discover and correct subconscious patterns.

It is as if taking a psychedelic temporarily "softens" a solid brain full of rigid pathological thought patterns and models into a more malleable one, allowing it to be reshaped before it solidifies again and its hierarchical structure reappears, but this time maybe slightly improved for the person's mental health.

Another simile of this process in sociopolitical terms would be to imagine the hierarchy of the brain as a highly stratified social class system with a bad authoritarian government that maintains a status quo that does not work well (DMN), hardly listening to the working classes (sensory networks and others), and oppressing them. In this scenario, the psychedelic experience would be the equivalent of a social revolt that seeks to break the system of hierarchies and social classes, and change the government, and even if it only achieves a temporary collapse of the system (and the previous social stratification), the government that is established again later will be something different from what it was before. It will have learned from the process and what it experienced and will listen more to social demands in the future.

It could be said that psychedelics expand consciousness by erasing the borders that our own ego imposes on us and allowing our models of the world to collapse, while mixing and updating with what surrounds them (us) at that moment, hence the paramount importance that these experiences are carried out with a clear intention, in controlled contexts and with adequate preparation of the patient—in other words, while taking very good care of the set and setting.

The reduction of activity in the DMN and the dissolution of the ego also reduce rumination, which is very present in most disorders, making it easier for us to stop being the center of the universe, living inside our heads, and for our problems to be relativized. We are then able to see them from a distance, with perspective, like an astronaut looking onto Earth and realizing the insignificance of their problems compared with the immensity of space.

This is combined with a subjective experience, which in good therapeutic conditions can be full of revelations, epiphanies, and new points of view. Since properly prepared psychedelic experiences allow us to facilitate new perspectives of the world and our problems, we can see them from afar, with fresh eyes, finding new meanings to things, new answers to the most basic questions related to our existence or the universe (such as the meaning of life), new purposes in life, which are often concealed under mental disorders such as depression or anxiety. Likewise, they allow us to review autobiographical content of a traumatic nature from a new perspective that allows it to be reprocessed and reframed, making great advances in the therapeutic process of various disorders such as PTSD or addictions.

In the words of Robin Carhart-Harris, former director of the Center for Psychedelic Research at Imperial College London:

The impact of successful psychedelic therapy is often one of revelation or epiphany. People speak about witnessing the "big picture," placing things in perspective, accessing deep insight about themselves and the world, releasing pent-up mental pain, feeling physically and emotionally recalibrated, clear-sighted, and equanimous. This is very different from people's descriptions of the effects of SSRIs (the most common antidepressants today), where a contrasting feeling of being emotionally muted is not uncommon.[13]

Many of these revelations may not have great therapeutic value later, but some do, and in order to reinforce and implement these new insights into life, in combination with this psychedelic-induced temporary neuroplasticity window, it is important to follow a process of psychological integration afterwards, as we will see later.

What some studies have found is that living a mystical experience during the psychedelic therapy session is what best predicts later improvement in a disorder, in other words, that the mystical experience is an important part of the therapeutic process. If two people get exactly the same dose, but one goes through that kind of experience and the other doesn't reach that level, the one who does is much more likely to have a lasting therapeutic result than the other.

Of course, all this will depend a lot on the person's set and setting, their intentions, and so on, and there is always the possibility of living a difficult experience, with anxiety and fear. This, although it does not usually last longer than a few hours, could produce negative changes if it is not well managed during and afterwards.

---

13. Robin Carhart-Harris, "We Can No Longer Ignore the Potential of Psychedelic Drugs to Treat Depression," *The Guardian* (June 8, 2020): online.

6

The Present and Future of Clinical Research with Psychedelic Drugs

PSYCHEDELIC-ASSISTED PSYCHOTHERAPY

As we have mentioned before, when we talk about psychedelic therapies, in most cases we are actually referring to a model known as psychedelic-assisted psychotherapy. Within the different models of psychedelic therapies, this is the one that currently seems to be offering the greatest therapeutic efficacy, safety, and efficiency.

This model combines classic elements of psychotherapy with some specific pharmacological interventions (sessions) of psychedelics under direct professional supervision, and a post-session integration process that allows subjects to continue working on those experiences. This model does not require the use of psychedelic substances on more than one or very few occasions, and its therapeutic effects are very long lasting.

There are several different ways in which psychedelic-assisted psychotherapy can be structured and it will depend on many factors, such as the psychedelic drug being used. At present, the most effective and efficient format to work with each substance and condition is not yet fully optimized, so it is possible that in the near future this therapeutic model will evolve along with the findings and the accumulation of new evidence that will maximize its results and safety, while also minimizing its cost in each case. This has led to some new trial designs in the last years with minimal or no psychotherapeutic intervention, just safety support, but the most common approach in the clinical research context so far is a therapeutic intervention divided into three blocks: screening and preparation, administration, and integration and follow-up; the administration and integration may be repeated within a certain period of time depending on the specific study protocol or the patient response to the treatment.

- Screening: Therapy usually begins with a screening or evaluation to rule out patients who may not be suitable for psychedelic treatment. Patients with a propensity for some psychiatric illnesses, such as bipolarity, psychotic disorders, or schizophrenia, or a family history of these, are usually excluded due to the serious risk of precipitating an episode. Also, people with heart problems, who are pregnant, or whose general physical health can bring about complications in the event of an emotionally intense experience are excluded.

- Preparation: Once it has been verified that the person does not have a condition or psychiatric disorder that could be especially dangerous for the consumption of psychedelics, work is carried out during a number of sessions to evaluate and prepare the patient for the psychedelic experience. In order to properly prepare the psychedelic experience, it is very important to work on the expectations for it (a common mantra for a good approach to the psychedelic journey is the famous "trust, let go, and be open" by William "Bill" Richards), define an intention that serves as an initial orientation during the session, strengthen the trust and bond between patients and the therapists who will accompany them during the administration of the psychedelic (usually a male and a female), as well as preparing for possible psychological difficulties that may occur during the session—such as the feeling of going crazy or dying—by using relaxation and coping techniques (for example, not running away from what frightens us, but facing it and asking, "What have you come to teach me?" and knowing that all is in our head and won't harm us). Also, relaxation techniques such as breathing are learned and tried beforehand in case of acute fear and anxiety showing up during the trip.

- Administration: When the patient is ready, the administration session is scheduled. Depending on the pathology and the psychedelic substance to be used, there are different ways to proceed, but the most common procedure is for sessions to start in the morning, a few hours after a very light breakfast. The accompanying therapists (usually a male and a female) and the patient go into a room that has been prepared and set for the session. In it, one last conversation is had, reminding the participant of the instructions ("trust, let go, and be open") and the intention for that session. The patient ingests the psychedelic compound and lies down to relax while waiting for its effects to start. Psychedelic sessions are non-directive and designed to invite introspection; to promote this, patients are asked to wear an eye mask. They also wear headphones with a specially selected playlist to accompany them throughout, thus facilitating the different phases of the session. Reaching the quality and intensity of a mystical experience[1] is usually correlated with better therapeutic results, so it is desirable.

- Integration: During the integration phase, the patient and psychotherapist work on all the material that has emerged during the administration session. This is the phase where most of the psychotherapy occurs. Sometimes, if the protocols of the study contemplate it (remember that most psychedelic-assisted psychotherapy work carried out today is in the context of clinical trials), the administration and integration sessions can be repeated after a few weeks, depending on how many are planned in the treatment protocol. The most common approach is to have two: one with a medium dose and another with a high dose, but lately single-dose protocols are very common too.

- Follow-up: This is a phase that occurs mostly in clinical research, and its function is to evaluate if the changes and therapeutic improvements produced during the administration session and integration work last and for how long. It also allows for detecting any relapses and evaluating if another psychedelic session is necessary.

---

1. A mystical experience is a very personal introspective experience where some kind of universal unity or transcendence of time and space is described.

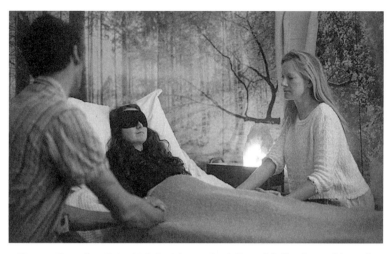

Recreation of a clinical trial with psychedelics with Dr. Jonny Martell,
Dr. Roberta Murphy, and Dr. Rosalind Watts at the Imperial Centre for
Psychedelic Research. Photo by Thomas Angus,
Imperial College London.

During the session, which can vary in length depending on the psychedelic used, interactions between therapists and patients are commonly limited to support if requested by the latter, holding hands and other comforting gestures, or accompanying them to the bathroom.

In the specific case of MDMA-assisted psychotherapy work, which is mostly applied in post-traumatic stress disorder, there is more freedom to interact with the patient and some psychotherapy work can be performed during the administration sessions (in the case of MDMA, there are usually three or four sessions).

Let's briefly see some of the results that psychedelic-assisted therapies are having in clinical research for different mental health conditions:

POST-TRAUMATIC STRESS DISORDER (PTSD)

One of the areas in which substances with psychedelic effects, and more specifically MDMA (ecstasy), are showing greater efficacy is in the treatment of post-traumatic stress disorder (PTSD). MDMA already concluded a few phase 3 clinical trials in the United States (the last phase before it is authorized for medical use), an initiative backed by MAPS (now led by its for-profit public benefit corporation [PBC] branch Lykos Therapeutics). After a first negative FDA evaluation in August 2024, Lykos Therapeutics will be running another phase 3 trial using MDMA to gain FDA authorization in the next few years. There is also some phase 2 research exploring the use of other psychedelics such as psilocybin or ketamine for PTSD (like those from Compass Pathways, Apex Labs, and Seelos Therapeutics).

Post-traumatic stress disorder is a mental health problem that develops in a person after experiencing or witnessing a traumatic event (such as war, assault, rape, accident, kidnapping). After having experienced this event, it is normal for the body to go into alert mode, characterized by fear reactions, release of certain hormones, and creating fight or flight responses like increased blood pressure, increased heart rate, rapid breathing, and pupil dilation. This response lasts for a while, even after the threat has already disappeared.

Normally, this reaction decreases over time so the person can return to a normal life, with the traumatic event gradually subsiding from present memory, without it becoming a stumbling block in their life. But there are also cases in which the person continues to suffer, reliving this event and reacting very intensely to it in the absence of the threat, even decades later, having enormous difficulties in resuming a normal life or a good quality of life. These people who remain chronically affected by trauma may be diagnosed with post-traumatic stress disorder.

The most common symptoms usually include re-experiencing the trauma in the form of flashbacks, nightmares, intrusive thoughts, avoidance strategies (such as avoiding places or objects that remind the event), being hypervigilant (insomnia, tension, anxiety, easily startled) and reactive. Also, some people may show cognitive or mood symptoms, such as feelings of guilt, problems with memory and concentration, depression, anxiety, or loss of interest in things.

Currently, this disorder affects many millions of people in the world. It occurs especially among those who have experienced natural disasters, violence, war, abuse, rape, or accidents. It is estimated that 7–12% of the population suffers from it to a greater or lesser extent, and that 60% of men and 50% of women have experienced at least one traumatic event in their lives. The successful treatment of this pathology is especially important, given that traumas are at the base of many mental illnesses, and that they are responsible for much disability, suffering, addictions, and deaths by suicide every year in the world.

Currently, this disorder is treated with psychotherapy combined with pharmacological interventions based on antidepressants (like the famous selective serotonin reuptake inhibitors, SSRIs, such as fluoxetine [Prozac]) and anxiolytics (like the well-known benzodiazepines, such as lorazepam [Orfidal]), or with therapies such as EMDR (Eye Movement Desensitization and Reprocessing).[2] Unfortunately, a significant percentage of people who suffer from this disorder do not manage to recover through the conventional treatments and become chronic treatment-resistant patients. It is in these type of patients that treatments with MDMA-assisted psychotherapy are being tested the most.

In this disorder, MDMA-assisted psychotherapy is proving to be extremely effective in patients who have not been able to recover through classic psychotherapy treatments combined with antidepressants and anxiolytics.

As we have seen in the previous chapter, there are many ways in which MDMA is a suitable substance for this. In addition to its psychedelic effects, MDMA reduces the activation of the amygdala, which is the area of the brain responsible for fear and the fight-or-flight response that accompanies it, allowing the patient to remember the traumatic event from a safe place, without suffering an excessive negative emotional response or fear. In addition, given its empathogen/entactogen effect, it helps the patient feel safe, trusting and sharing their experience more easily with the therapist. It also facilitates self-compassion, eliminating the feelings of guilt or responsibility often associated with this type of trauma. Likewise, the neuroplasticity derived from the activation of the 5-HT2a neuroreceptors

---

2. EMDR is a form of psychotherapy that is particularly effective in treating post-traumatic stress disorder and other trauma-related conditions. EMDR involves the patient recalling distressing events while simultaneously undergoing bilateral sensory input, such as side-to-side eye movements, which is believed to help process and reduce the emotional impact of traumatic memories.

allows this new way of understanding and evaluating the traumatic event to be established more easily, as if fear were unlearned.

Several clinical trials have been conducted in recent years exploring this. We will discuss some examples in the following pages.

MDMA-Assisted Therapy for Severe PTSD: A Randomized, Double-Blind, Placebo-Controlled Phase 3 Study

Jennifer M. Mitchell et al., from *Nature Medicine* 27, no. 6 (June 2021): 1025–33.

This study was a double blind,[3] placebo-controlled[4] clinical trial to test the efficacy and safety of MDMA-assisted therapy for the treatment of patients with severe PTSD. After three preparation sessions, ninety PTSD patients (suffering from the condition for an average of fourteen years) received MDMA or placebo therapy, followed by nine integration sessions.

PTSD symptoms (measured with the CAPS-V PTSD Scale), and functional impairment (measured with the Sheehan Disability Scale, SDS), were assessed at baseline and two months after the last experimental session. MDMA was found to induce a significant and robust attenuation in the CAPS-V PTSD scale score compared to placebo and significantly reduce the total SDS score. The mean change in CAPS-V PTSD scores in participants who completed treatment was a reduction

---

3. Neither researchers nor patients know who receives MDMA and who receives a placebo, until the end of the study.

4. A placebo is a substance that lacks pharmacological action for the treatment of a pathology, but can produce an effect by suggestion if the person taking it is convinced that it is really a drug with effects (called "expectancy"). Normally clinical trials are done by comparing the effect of the drug being studied with a placebo, for which it is necessary that neither patients nor therapists know which is the placebo and which is the active drug (this is called "double blind") until the end of the study, for which both have the same appearance, taste, and shape; if both turn out to have similar effects or effectiveness, it means that the drug is not really doing anything beyond the placebo effect itself and therefore its effectiveness and pharmaceutical development is discarded.

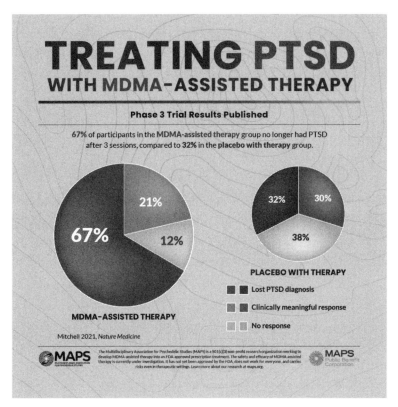

Graph representing the results of the study in the treatment group versus the control group. Sourced via MAPS. (See also color plate 12.)

of 24.4 points in the MDMA group versus a reduction of 13.9 points in the placebo group.

Sixty-seven percent of participants who received three sessions of MDMA-assisted psychotherapy no longer met diagnostic criteria for PTSD (versus 32% achieved by placebo therapy), and 88% experienced a clinically relevant reduction in symptoms (versus 62% who improved with placebo therapy).

MDMA did not induce adverse events of abuse potential, suicidality, or heart problems.

These data indicated that, compared to normal therapy combined with an inactive placebo, MDMA-assisted therapy is highly effective in people with severe PTSD and the treatment is safe and well tolerated, even in those with comorbidities.

MDMA-Assisted Therapy for Moderate to Severe PTSD: A Randomized, Placebo-Controlled Phase 3 Trial

Jennifer M. Mitchell et al., from *Nature Medicine* 29
(September 14, 2023): 2473–2480.

This study aimed to determine how effective and safe MDMA-assisted therapy (MDMA-AT) is for people with moderate to severe post-traumatic stress disorder (PTSD). The study was a double-blind, randomized design, meaning neither the participants nor the researchers knew who was receiving MDMA or a placebo.

The study involved 104 people with PTSD (53 received MDMA-AT, 51 received placebo with therapy); 26.9% had moderate PTSD and 73.1% had severe PTSD.

- CAPS-5 scores: Participants who received MDMA-AT showed a significant reduction in PTSD symptoms, with an average decrease of 23.7 points. Those in the placebo group had a smaller reduction, averaging 14.8 points.
- SDS scores: Functional impairment decreased more in the MDMA-AT group, with an average reduction of 3.3 points, compared to a 2.1-point reduction in the placebo group.
- Safety: Seven participants experienced severe side effects (5 in the MDMA-AT group and 2 in the placebo group), but there were no deaths or serious adverse events.

MDMA-assisted therapy significantly reduced PTSD symptoms and improved daily functioning in a diverse group of participants with moderate to severe PTSD. The treatment was generally well tolerated. Further research could solidify MDMA-AT as a viable option for PTSD treatment.

BREAKTHROUGH FOR TRAUMA TREATMENT: SAFETY
AND EFFICACY OF MDMA-ASSISTED PSYCHOTHERAPY
COMPARED TO PAROXETINE AND SERTRALINE
Allison A. Feduccia et al., from *Frontiers in Psychiatry* 10
(September 12, 2019): 650.

Paroxetine and sertraline, both SSRIs, are commonly used to treat PTSD, but research has shown that their effectiveness is only modest compared to placebos. In contrast, six phase 2 trials found that MDMA-assisted psychotherapy had a much greater impact on reducing PTSD symptoms. The studies showed that MDMA's effect was about twice as strong as paroxetine's and three times stronger than sertraline's. Specifically, MDMA treatment led to a 26.2-point improvement in CAPS-IV Total PTSD Severity scores, compared to 6–14 points for paroxetine and 6.8–9.8 points for sertraline. Additionally, MDMA's benefits appeared more quickly—within 3–5 days—whereas SSRIs can take several weeks to show effects. The positive impact of MDMA therapy also lasted for at least a year.

Interestingly, while sertraline was only significantly effective in women, MDMA worked equally well for both men and women. Comparing the data from these studies, the Multidisciplinary Association for Psychedelic Studies (MAPS) concluded that MDMA-assisted therapy offers a significant improvement over current medications in terms of both safety and effectiveness. The studies also showed lower dropout rates for MDMA therapy compared to SSRIs, partly because MDMA is administered in a controlled setting, reducing the risk of overdose, withdrawal symptoms, or other complications.

DEPRESSION AND ANXIETY

Depression and anxiety are two of the conditions for which substances with psychedelic effects (especially pure or classic psychedelics such as psilocybin) are showing greater efficacy and are closer to being authorized for medical use. In fact, there are a lot of companies currently running phase 2–3 clinical trials with psilocybin (including Compass Pathways, Usona Institute, Braxia, GH Research, and Cybin), the Compass Pathways trials being already well underway. But there is also a lot of research into the use of esketamine (a purified form of ketamine containing only one of its enantiomers), which has already been licensed for the treatment of treatment-resistant depression and is marketed under the name Spravato by Janssen (from Johnson & Johnson).

Depression is a mental illness that can be attributed to various causes (psychological, genetic, environmental, biological) but that usually manifests as a deep feeling of emptiness, sadness, lack of motivation and interest, fatigue, anhedonia (lack of pleasure), trouble sleeping or excessive sleepiness, loss of or excessive appetite, and, in more severe cases, may be accompanied by the desire to disappear and suicidal ideations.

Currently, major depressive disorder is a disease that affects more than 300 million people in the world, being the leading cause of disability, increasing the relative risk of death by 1.7 times compared to the general population in the United States. Approximately 10% of the adult U.S. population has been diagnosed with depression in the past year, and the annual cost is estimated at around $210 billion dollars.

Nowadays, it is mainly treated with psychotherapy combined with pharmacological interventions such as antidepressants and anxiolytics, but these substances have limited efficacy and also side effects that make it difficult for some patients to adhere to treatment. Although this treatment reduces depressive symptoms and even achieves remission in many patients, approximately 30% to 50% do not respond at all, and 10% to 30% do not obtain more improvement than if they were given a placebo,[5] which means they are not obtaining benefits from the pharmacological treatment.

In depression, psychedelic-assisted psychotherapy is proving to be

---

5. Bradley N. Gaynes et al., "What Did STAR*D Teach Us? Results from a Large-Scale, Practical, Clinical Trial for Patients with Depression," *Psychiatric Services* 60, no. 11 (November 2009): 1439–45.

quite effective in patients who have not managed to recover through classical treatments, like psychotherapy combined with antidepressants and anxiolytics.

As we have seen in the previous chapter, there are many reasons why psychedelics are suitable substances for this and, unlike SSRI (selective serotonin reuptake inhibitors) antidepressants, they do not focus on covering up symptoms or blunting emotions. Rather, they allow the person to find and confront the underlying cause(s) of their condition, also allowing a window of neuroplasticity that can facilitate lasting changes in the disorder, in the perception of oneself, and in the perception of the world.

Likewise, they help patients with terminal illnesses to accept their illness, lose the paralyzing fear of death, and find meaning and enjoyment in their last months or years of life, even declaring that they feel "greater clarity and confidence about their personal values and priorities, and a renewed or enhanced recognition of the intrinsic meaning and value of life."[6]

In recent years, the results of several clinical trials exploring these therapeutic uses of psilocybin have been published. We will now discuss some of them.

SINGLE-DOSE PSILOCYBIN FOR A TREATMENT-RESISTANT EPISODE OF MAJOR DEPRESSION

Guy M. Goodwin et al., from *New England Journal of Medicine* 387, no. 18 (November 2022): 1637–1648.

In this study, researchers tested how effective a synthetic form of psilocybin is for adults with depression that hasn't responded to other treatments. The study included 233 participants who were given a single dose of either 25 mg, 10 mg, or 1 mg (as a control) of psilocybin, along with psychological support. The main goal was to see how much their depression scores changed after 3 weeks, using a standard scale called

---

6. Ira Byock, "Taking Psychedelics Seriously," *Journal of Palliative Medicine* 21, no. 4 (April 2018): 417–21.

the Montgomery–Åsberg Depression Rating Scale (MADRS), where higher scores mean more severe depression.

Here's what they found:

- The group that received 25 mg of psilocybin showed the most significant improvement, with their depression scores dropping by an average of 12 points.
- The group that received 10 mg had a smaller improvement, with an average drop of 7.9 points.
- The control group (1 mg) had the least improvement, with an average drop of 5.4 points.

When comparing the groups, the 25 mg dose was much more effective than the 1 mg dose. However, the difference between the 10 mg and 1 mg doses was not statistically significant. About 77% of the participants experienced minor side effects like headaches, nausea, and dizziness. There were also reports of suicidal thoughts or behaviors across all dose groups.

In conclusion, a single 25 mg dose of psilocybin significantly reduced depression scores more than a 1 mg dose over three weeks, but it came with some side effects. More extensive and longer studies are needed to compare psilocybin with existing treatments and to further evaluate its safety and effectiveness.

SINGLE-DOSE PSILOCYBIN-ASSISTED THERAPY IN MAJOR DEPRESSIVE DISORDER: A PLACEBO-CONTROLLED, DOUBLE-BLIND, RANDOMISED CLINICAL TRIAL
Robin von Rotz et al., from *eClinical Medicine* 56 (February 2023): 101809.

In this study, 52 participants with major depressive disorder, but no severe physical health issues, were randomly assigned to receive either a single, moderate dose of psilocybin (0.215 mg/kg body weight) or a placebo. Both groups also received psychological support. Depression severity was measured using the Montgomery–Åsberg Depression Rating Scale (MADRS) and the Beck Depression Inventory (BDI), from the start of the study to 14 days after the treatment.

These were the findings:

- Symptom reduction: Participants who received psilocybin showed a significant decrease in depression symptoms. Their MADRS scores dropped by an average of 13 points, which was much greater than the reduction seen in the placebo group.
- Remission rates: In the psilocybin group, 54% of participants (14 out of 26) met the criteria for remission according to MADRS.
- Safety: No serious adverse events were reported.

The researchers interpreted that a single, moderate dose of psilocybin significantly reduced depressive symptoms for at least two weeks compared to a placebo. These promising results suggest that further large-scale and longer-term studies are needed to refine this treatment approach.

EFFECTS OF PSILOCYBIN-ASSISTED THERAPY ON MAJOR DEPRESSIVE DISORDER: A RANDOMIZED CLINICAL TRIAL

Alan K. Davis et al., from *JAMA Psychiatry* 78, no. 5 (May 1, 2021): 481–89.

In this Johns Hopkins University study, a group of 24 people who had been suffering from depression for an average of more than 20 years, with no history of psychotic disorder, suicide attempts, or serious hospitalization were given 2 doses of psilocybin, first 20 mg and then a second dose of 30 mg.

After the first psilocybin session, 71% of patients reported decreases of more than 50% in their depression symptoms.

After the second psilocybin session, 71% of patients reported decreases of more than 50% in their depression symptoms.

After the first week, 58% of the participants were in remission (their symptoms were so reduced that they no longer met diagnostic criteria for depression).

At 4 weeks, the patients were followed up, and 54% of the participants were still in remission (their symptoms were greatly reduced).

The conclusion of this study is that psilocybin-assisted psychotherapy produces large, rapid, and persistent antidepressant effects over time in patients with chronic depression resistant to conventional treatment. Adverse effects that were reported were not serious and were transient, such as mild to moderate headache and challenging emotions, which were limited to the time of the session.

However, there were some limitations of this study, like the small number of participants, the absence of a placebo group (although there was a control group), and the exclusion of participants with more severe forms of the disease that included previous suicide attempts.

EFFICACY AND SAFETY OF PSILOCYBIN-ASSISTED TREATMENT FOR MAJOR DEPRESSIVE DISORDER: PROSPECTIVE 12-MONTH FOLLOW-UP

Natalie Gukasyan et al., from *Journal of Psychopharmacology* 36, no. 2 (February 2022): 151–58.

In this study, researchers observed significant reductions in depression scores at multiple points—1, 3, 6, and 12 months—following psilocybin-assisted therapy. One year after treatment, 75% of participants continued to show a strong response, defined as a reduction in depression scores by more than half, while 58% were in remission. Importantly, there were no serious side effects linked to psilocybin during the follow-up period, and participants did not report using psilocybin outside the study.

The study also found that participants who rated their sessions as personally significant or spiritually meaningful tended to report greater well-being after 12 months. However, these experiences did not directly correlate with improvements in depression.

Overall, the findings suggest that psilocybin-assisted therapy can provide lasting antidepressant effects for many patients, with benefits that extend for at least a year after just a few treatment sessions. This highlights the potential of psilocybin as a powerful and enduring treatment option for depression.

> ## PSILOCYBIN PRODUCES SUBSTANTIAL AND SUSTAINED DECREASES IN DEPRESSION AND ANXIETY IN PATIENTS WITH LIFE-THREATENING CANCER: A DOUBLE-BLIND RANDOMIZED TRIAL
>
> Roland R. Griffiths et al., from *Journal of Psychopharmacology* 30, no. 12 (December 2016): 1181–97.

In a study conducted by the Johns Hopkins University team, 51 patients with life-threatening cancer and accompanying depression or anxiety were given either a substantial dose of psilocybin (20 mg to 30 mg) or a very low, almost imperceptible dose as a placebo (1 mg to 3 mg). Throughout the study, the moods, attitudes, and behaviors of the participants were closely monitored by themselves, the staff, and people from their communities.

The results showed that those who received the higher doses of psilocybin experienced significant reductions in depression and anxiety. These improvements were also accompanied by an enhanced quality of life, a greater sense of meaning, increased optimism, and less fear of death. Remarkably, these positive effects were still evident six months after the treatment, with around 80% of participants continuing to show significant reductions in depression and anxiety.

Participants also reported feeling better about life and themselves, with improvements in mood, relationships, and spirituality. More than 80% of them noted a moderate or greater increase in their overall well-being and life satisfaction. These improvements were also confirmed by observations from their communities.

The study further explored the connection between the intensity of mystical experiences during the sessions and the therapeutic outcomes, finding that these experiences contributed to the positive effects. Importantly, there were no serious or lasting negative side effects linked to psilocybin. The most common side effects were mild and temporary, including psychological discomfort, anxiety, and headaches, all of which were resolved by the end of the session.

This study highlights the potential of psilocybin to significantly improve mental health and well-being in patients facing severe illness, with effects that can last for months.

RAPID AND SUSTAINED SYMPTOM REDUCTION FOLLOWING PSILOCYBIN TREATMENT FOR ANXIETY AND DEPRESSION IN PATIENTS WITH LIFE-THREATENING CANCER: A RANDOMIZED CONTROLLED TRIAL

Stephen Ross et al., from *Journal of Psychopharmacology* 30, no. 12 (December 2016): 1165–80.

In this study, 29 cancer patients experiencing anxiety and depression were treated with either a single dose of psilocybin (0.3 mg/kg) or niacin (which served as a placebo), both combined with psychotherapy. The trial was double-blind and placebo-controlled, ensuring that neither the participants nor the researchers knew which treatment was given until after the study.

The results were striking. Psilocybin led to immediate and significant improvements in anxiety and depression, along with reduced feelings of hopelessness and a lack of motivation. Patients also reported better spiritual well-being and an improved quality of life. Remarkably, these benefits lasted for at least 6.5 months, with 60% to 80% of participants still experiencing substantial reductions in anxiety and depression at follow-up. The treatment also helped sustain a better outlook on life and death.

The study found that the therapeutic effects of psilocybin were strongly linked to the mystical experiences reported by participants during the sessions. Overall, the findings suggest that a single moderate dose of psilocybin, when paired with psychotherapy, can provide rapid, powerful, and enduring relief from anxiety and depression in cancer patients.

LONG-TERM FOLLOW-UP OF PSILOCYBIN-ASSISTED PSYCHOTHERAPY FOR PSYCHIATRIC AND EXISTENTIAL DISTRESS IN PATIENTS WITH LIFE-THREATENING CANCER

Gabrielle I. Agin-Liebes et al., from *Journal of Psychopharmacology* 34, no. 2 (February 2020): 155–66.

This study followed up on the previous Ross study 4.5 years later to assess the long-term effects of psilocybin-assisted therapy in cancer patients. The results showed that the reductions in anxiety, depression, hopelessness, lack of motivation, and death anxiety observed in the original study were largely maintained over time. Effect sizes within the group were significant, with around 60–80% of participants still experiencing clinically significant relief from depression or anxiety after 4.5 years.

Nearly all participants reported that the psilocybin-assisted therapy had led to positive life changes, describing it as one of the most meaningful and spiritually significant experiences of their lives. These findings suggest that psilocybin-assisted psychotherapy could offer lasting benefits for those dealing with cancer-related psychological distress. However, due to the crossover design of the original study, the ability to draw definitive conclusions about the therapy's efficacy is limited.

EFFICACY AND SAFETY OF INTRANASAL ESKETAMINE ADJUNCTIVE TO ORAL ANTIDEPRESSANT THERAPY IN TREATMENT-RESISTANT DEPRESSION: A RANDOMIZED CLINICAL TRIAL

Ella J. Daly et al., from *JAMA Psychiatry* 75, no. 2 (February 2018): 139–48.

In 2019, esketamine, a variant of the ketamine molecule, was approved in the U.S. and Europe for treating depression, marking it as the first psychedelic-like substance authorized for mental health therapy when used alongside traditional antidepressants. The Daly study explored its potential in a phase 2, double-blind, placebo-controlled trial involving

67 patients with treatment-resistant depression. These patients were randomly assigned to receive either a placebo or esketamine at doses of 28 mg, 56 mg, or 84 mg, administered twice a week, while continuing their existing antidepressant medication.

The study's main goal was to measure changes in depression symptoms using the Montgomery–Åsberg Depression Rating Scale (MADRS) by day 8. The results showed that esketamine led to greater reductions in depression scores compared to the placebo, with higher doses showing more significant improvements (28 mg: a reduction of 4.2 points; 56 mg: a reduction of 6.3 points; 84 mg: a reduction of 9.0 points). This antidepressant effect appeared to last, with a 7.2-point reduction even as the dosing frequency was decreased in the study's final phase.

However, 7% of patients (4 out of 56) who received esketamine experienced adverse effects, such as fainting, headaches, dissociative symptoms, and ectopic pregnancy, leading to their withdrawal from the study.

Overall, the study found that esketamine provided a rapid and dose-dependent antidepressant effect, which persisted for over two months with reduced dosing.

Another interesting study to consider regarding depression and psychedelic-assisted therapy is "Trial of Psilocybin versus Escitalopram for Depression."[7]

ADDICTIONS

The use of psychedelic substances for the treatment of addictions is currently being explored. These are mainly for substance addictions (substance use disorders), although they may also show potential for behavioral addictions. In the treatment of addictions to substances such as alcohol, tobacco, heroin, or cocaine, the psychedelics that are being explored the most are psilocybin, ibogaine, MDMA, DMT (normally in the form of ayahuasca), and LSD.

---

7. Robin Carhart-Harris et al., "Trial of Psilocybin versus Escitalopram for Depression," *The New England Journal of Medicine* 384, no. 15 (April 15, 2021): 1402–11.

Addictions, whether to substances or behavioral (for example, gambling, sex, social networks, shopping, or food) represent a huge public health problem today. Substance use disorders affect hundreds of millions of people globally, accounting for the loss of more than 130 million DALYs (disability-adjusted life years) in 2016. Today, it is one of the main causes of the 11.8 million annual deaths related to alcohol, tobacco, and other drugs.

The diagnostic manual of mental disorders, in its latest edition (*DSM-5*), defines substance use disorder as a pathological pattern of behaviors related to the persistent use of drugs (including alcohol) despite substantial harm and adverse consequences. The essential feature of substance use disorders is the association of cognitive, behavioral, and physiological symptoms that indicate that the person continues to use the substance despite significant problems related to it. The diagnosis can be made on ten classes of substances that have been included in the *DSM-5*, except for caffeine: "For some substances, these symptoms are less conspicuous, and not even all symptoms occur (e.g., withdrawal symptoms are not specified in phencyclidine, other hallucinogen, or inhalant use disorder). An important feature of substance use disorder is the underlying change in brain circuits that persists after detoxification, and that occurs especially in people with severe disorders. The behavioral effects of these brain changes are shown in repeated relapses and intense cravings when the person is exposed to drug-related stimuli."[8] This definition could be expanded in the coming years with the inclusion of criteria for addictions without substance or smoking, which would drastically increase the number of people who would meet its diagnostic criteria.

Unfortunately, current mental health treatments do not achieve sufficient efficacy rates to counteract or alleviate this increase in prevalence, and their majority treatment model is in question. It is especially in the field of addictions where there are more populations of chronic

---

8. American Psychiatric Association, *Diagnostic and Statistical Manual of Mental Disorders*, 5th ed. (Washington, DC: American Psychiatric Association, 2013); see pages 483–484.

patients resistant to such treatments or with difficulties in adherence. The effectiveness of these treatments involves a high consumption of economic, health, and human resources, a cost that in many cases is assumed by the public health systems and by the patients themselves, together with the great productivity loss caused by the disorder. In addition, these are treatments with multiple side effects and health risks derived from the chronic use of psychotropic drugs such as antidepressants, anxiolytics, or antipsychotics; without forgetting the complex pharmacological interactions with other drugs, often toxic, as well as the risk of using these substances for suicide purposes.

These conventional therapies, which have hardly evolved in recent decades, are proving insufficient to contain this mental health epidemic, while other areas of medicine and health have experienced a very important and exponential evolution in recent years.

Addictions, like depression or PTSD, manifest psychologically through rigid patterns of thought and behavior, and it is common to find that they developed as a response to voids or traumas. That is why they are a strong candidate for psychedelic-assisted psychotherapy. In fact, this model of treatment emerged precisely in the work with people with alcoholism problems in the late 1950s.

In recent years, several clinical trials have been carried out exploring this field.[9] Let's look at a few important ones.

PERCENTAGE OF HEAVY DRINKING DAYS FOLLOWING PSILOCYBIN-ASSISTED PSYCHOTHERAPY VS PLACEBO IN THE TREATMENT OF ADULT PATIENTS WITH ALCOHOL USE DISORDER: A RANDOMIZED CLINICAL TRIAL

Michael P. Bogenschutz et al., from *JAMA Psychiatry* 79, no. 10 (August 2022): 953–962.

---

9. Anton Gomez-Escolar et al., "Current Perspectives on the Clinical Research and Medicalization of Psychedelic Drugs for Addiction Treatments: Safety, Efficacy, Limitations and Challenges," *CNS Drugs* 38, no. 9 (2024): 771–89.

This study aimed to determine if two high-dose psilocybin sessions could reduce heavy drinking days in people with Alcohol Use Disorder (AUD) receiving psychotherapy, compared to a placebo with psychotherapy.

This double-blind, randomized clinical trial included participants undergoing 12 weeks of structured psychotherapy. They were randomly assigned to receive either psilocybin or diphenhydramine (placebo) during 2 medication sessions at weeks 4 and 8. The effects were monitored for 32 weeks post-treatment. The trial took place at 2 academic centers in the U.S. Participants were adults aged 25 to 65 with a diagnosis of alcohol dependence and at least 4 heavy drinking days in the month prior to the study. Exclusion criteria included major psychiatric disorders, other drug use disorders, certain medical conditions, or ongoing AUD treatment.

Participants received either psilocybin (25 mg initially and 25–40 mg later) or diphenhydramine (50 mg initially and 50–100 mg later). Psychotherapy included motivational enhancement therapy and cognitive behavioral therapy.

The primary measure was the percentage of heavy drinking days, assessed over the 32-week period following the first medication dose through interviews.

Out of 95 participants, those in the psilocybin group had an average of 9.7% heavy drinking days, while the diphenhydramine group had 23.6%, a difference of 13.9%. The psilocybin group also showed lower daily alcohol consumption. No serious adverse events were reported in the psilocybin group.

Psilocybin combined with psychotherapy significantly reduced heavy drinking days compared to the placebo. These findings support further research into psilocybin-assisted treatment for AUD.

PILOT STUDY OF THE 5-HT2AR AGONIST PSILOCYBIN IN THE TREATMENT OF TOBACCO ADDICTION

Matthew W. Johnson et al., from *Journal of Psychopharmacology* 28, no. 11 (November 2014): 983–92.

This pilot study explored the effects of moderate (20 mg) and high (30 mg) doses of psilocybin as part of a 15-week cognitive behavioral therapy program aimed at helping people quit smoking. The study involved 15 healthy participants who had smoked an average of 19 cigarettes per day for 31 years and had previously made 6 attempts to quit.

The results were promising: 12 out of 15 participants (80%) successfully quit smoking and remained smoke-free for at least 6 months after the treatment. This success rate is significantly higher than the typical rates of less than 35% seen with other behavioral or pharmacological treatments.

While the open-label design of the study means that definitive conclusions about psilocybin's effectiveness can't be made, the findings suggest that psilocybin could be a promising addition to existing smoking cessation therapies.

LONG-TERM FOLLOW-UP OF PSILOCYBIN-FACILITATED SMOKING CESSATION

Matthew W. Johnson, Albert Garcia-Romeu, and Roland R. Griffiths, from *The American Journal of Drug and Alcohol Abuse* 43, no. 1 (January 2017): 55–60.

At 12 and 16 months, the follow-up of the participants in the previous study by Matthew Johnson found that, at 12 months, 67% of the participants were still smoke-free, and at 16 months it was confirmed that 60% were still smoke-free. 86.7% of the participants rated their experiences with psilocybin among the 5 most personally and spiritually significant experiences of their lives. Thus, these results suggest that, in the context of a structured treatment program, psilocybin holds great promise for promoting long-term tobacco abstinence.

CESSATION AND REDUCTION IN ALCOHOL CONSUMPTION AND MISUSE AFTER PSYCHEDELIC USE

Albert Garcia-Romeu et al., from *Journal of Psychopharmacology* 33, no. 9 (September 2019): 1088–1101.

This study reports the findings of an anonymous, online survey of people with prior alcohol use disorder (AUD), but who reported cessation or reduction of use after psychedelic use in non-clinical settings.

The number of people who completed the survey was 343. The participants reported a median of 7 years of problematic alcohol use (72% met retrospective criteria for severe AUD) prior to the psychedelic experience, to which they attributed the reduction in alcohol use. Most reported a significant reduction after taking a moderate or high dose of LSD (38%) or psilocybin (36%).

After the psychedelic experience, 83% no longer met diagnostic criteria for AUD, the disorder had remitted. Participants rated their psychedelic experience as highly significant and "insightful," and for 28% it was the changes in life priorities or values associated with the psychedelic experience that facilitated the reduction in alcohol misuse. A higher psychedelic dose, the sensation of insight, mystical-type effects, and the personal meaning of these experiences were the elements that were related to a greater reduction in alcohol consumption, facilitating the control of previous consumption and associated distress.

Although the results of an online survey are unable to prove causality or rule out a placebo effect, they suggest that psychedelic use could lead to cessation or reduction of problem drinking, supporting further investigation of psychedelic-assisted treatments for AUD.

LYSERGIC ACID DIETHYLAMIDE (LSD) FOR ALCOHOLISM: META-ANALYSIS OF RANDOMIZED CONTROLLED TRIALS

Teri S. Krebs and Pål-Ørjan Johansen, from *Journal of Psychopharmacology* 26, no. 7 (July 2012): 994–1002.

This meta-analysis of randomized controlled trials assessed the clinical efficacy of LSD in the treatment of alcoholism. Six trials meeting all criteria were included, with a total of 536 participants.

Of the patients who took LSD as part of their treatment, 59% had less alcohol abuse compared to 38% of those who received the placebo. Those people who took LSD also reported greater alcohol withdrawal.

This effect was maintained at six months after treatment, but after a year, the difference between those who had taken LSD and those who had not taken LSD was no longer significant.

A single dose of LSD, in the context of various alcoholism treatment programs, was associated with decreased alcohol abuse.

Another interesting study to consider regarding addictions and psychedelic-assisted therapy is "Psilocybin-Assisted Treatment for Alcohol Dependence: A Proof-of-Concept Study."[10]

NEURODEGENERATIVE DISEASES, LONG COVID, AND NEUROREHABILITATION

The research field of possible psychedelic applications in the treatment of neurodegenerative diseases, such as dementia, Alzheimer's, or Parkinson's, or to accelerate learning or neurorehabilitation, is still in the realm of speculation and in the phase of preliminary studies. More so when talking about the potential therapeutic applications in new diseases like the recently described neurological long COVID that seems to include, among many other things, brain alterations comparable to other neurodegenerative diseases.

Neurodegenerative diseases, and especially those associated with age, are becoming more frequent in our societies as a result of increased life expectancy, aging, and various environmental, infectious, and cultural factors related to modern life.

In recent years, it has been discovered[11] that many substances with

---

10. Michael P. Bogenschutz et al., "Psilocybin-Assisted Treatment for Alcohol Dependence: A Proof-of-Concept Study," *Journal of Psychopharmacology* 29, no. 3 (March 2015): 289–99.

11. Cato M. H. deVos, Natasha L. Mason, and Kim P. C. Kuypers, "Psychedelics and Neuroplasticity: A Systematic Review Unraveling the Biological Underpinnings of Psychedelics," *Frontiers in Psychiatry* 12 (September 2021): 724606. See also Maximiliano V. Vargas, Lee E. Dunlap, Chunyang Dong, Samuel J. Carter, Robert J. Tombari, Shekib A. Jami, Lindsay P. Cameron, Seona D. Patel, Joseph J. Hennessey, Hannah N. Saeger, John D. McCorvy, John A. Gray, Lin Tian, and David E. Olson, "Psychedelics Promote Neuroplasticity through the Activation of Intracellular 5-HT2A Receptors," *Science* 379, no. 6633 (February 2023): 700–706.

psychedelic properties have the ability to induce neuroplasticity (facilitate the neural networks of the brain to change, adapt, and thus facilitate learning), synaptogenesis (the formation of new synapses or connections between neurons), and neurogenesis (the formation of new neurons in specific areas of the brain). In addition, psychedelics have been shown to increase several neuronal growth factors, such as brain-derived neurotrophic growth factor (BDNF) or nerve growth factor (NGF), and have anti-inflammatory effects at the neuronal level.

These findings open the door to the investigation of possible psychedelic use to counter neuronal aging and in neurodegenerative diseases, which are characterized by the death of neurons or loss of synapses, or also in situations that require the need to accelerate the readaptation of the brain, such as neurorehabilitation or learning processes in situations of neuronal damage, traumatic brain injuries, strokes, infections, or other.

Titles from study publications that showed promise in this regard and that can open the door to future trials in humans include:

The alkaloids of *Banisteriopsis caapi*, the plant source of the Amazonian hallucinogen ayahuasca, stimulate adult neurogenesis in vitro[12]

N,N-dimethyltryptamine compound found in the hallucinogenic tea ayahuasca, regulates adult neurogenesis in vitro and in vivo[13]

A single dose of psilocybin increases synaptic density and decreases 5-HT receptor density in the pig brain[14]

Psilocybin induces rapid and persistent growth of dendritic spines in the frontal cortex in vivo[15]

Low doses of LSD acutely increase BDNF blood plasma levels in healthy volunteers[16]

---

12. Jose A. Morales-García et al., from *Scientific Reports* 7, no. 1 (July 2017): 5309.
13. Jose A. Morales-Garcia et al., from *Translational Psychiatry*, 2020.
14. Nakul Ravi Raval et al., from *International Journal of Molecular Sciences* 22, no. 2 (January 2021).
15. Ling-Xiao Shao et al., from *Neuron* 109, no. 16 (August 2021): 2535–44.
16. Nadia R. P. W. Hutten et al., from *ACS Pharmacology & Translational Science* 4, no. 2 (April 2021): 461–66.

BEHAVIOR CHANGE

Another possibility that is speculated, based on several anecdotal reports, is to use psychedelics as tools to facilitate the change of habits, fundamentally those that may be more dangerous to health or society.

Through the combination of certain therapeutic interventions in improving habits, such as cognitive behavioral therapy or motivational interviewing, today the use of psychedelics could increase their efficacy and durability when it comes to promoting the improvement of diet, exercise, exposure to nature, and mindfulness or stress reduction practices, all of which can contribute to better health and physical and psychological well-being.[17]

COUPLES THERAPY AND
CONFLICT RESOLUTION

An important potential use of psychedelics, primarily MDMA, is in the resolution of conflicts in various fields. This use was explored mainly in the field of couples therapy in the 1970s and 1980s. There is clinical experience and some studies on the subject.

In therapeutic contexts, MDMA facilitates communication, empathy, understanding, and forgiveness. It reduces the negative interpretation of ourselves and others, the processing of negative emotions, and it reduces the reactivity and the defenses that can arise during a conflict.

In this regard, preliminary clinical studies, both specific and in combination with other diagnoses, especially post-traumatic stress disorder,[18] have been carried out with promising results.[19]

---

17. Pedro J. Teixeira et al., "Psychedelics and Health Behaviour Change," *Journal of Psychopharmacology* 36, no. 1 (January 2022): 12–19.
18. Candice M. Monson et al., "MDMA-Facilitated Cognitive-Behavioural Conjoint Therapy for Posttraumatic Stress Disorder: An Uncontrolled Trial," *European Journal of Psychotraumatology* 11, no. 1 (December 2020): 1840123.
19. Anne C. Wagner et al., "Relational and Growth Outcomes Following Couples Therapy with MDMA for PTSD," *Frontiers in Psychiatry* 12 (June 2021): 702838.

Likewise, its use is being explored in the context of other conflicts, such as the Palestinian-Israeli one, where some studies are obtaining very interesting results.[20]

MICRODOSING

In recent years, a practice has become popular that champions the use of psychedelics in very low doses and repeatedly throughout the week, following different dosage models that I will explain. According to its advocates, it can improve concentration, productivity (like nootropics),[21] creativity, mood, well-being, and even symptoms of depression, anxiety, PTSD, attention-deficit/hyperactivity disorder (ADHD), obsessive-compulsive disorder (OCD), and more.

Microdosing became popular after the publication of Jim Fadiman's book *The Psychedelic Explorer's Guide*.[22] In this book, he wrote of this practice, which consists of taking very low doses in the range of one tenth of the normal active dose of a psychedelic (the usual range of these microdoses is usually between one twelfth and one eighth) at the start of the day, as if it were coffee, and then carrying out normal daily activities. For example, in the case of LSD, the conventional active dose is 100 micrograms. When microdosing, a dose would fall in the range of 8 to 12 micrograms, normally 10 micrograms.

This practice is not practiced daily, but rather in the form of a scheduled protocol. There are several, but the most popular are:

• The Fadiman protocol, which alternates one day of intake with two days of rest.

---

20. Leor Roseman et al., "Relational Processes in Ayahuasca Groups of Palestinians and Israelis," *Frontiers in Pharmacology* 12 (May 2021): 607529.

21. A nootropic is a substance that is claimed to enhance cognitive functions such as memory, creativity, focus, and overall brain function. These substances can be natural or synthetic and are often referred to as "smart drugs" or cognitive enhancers.

22. James Fadiman, *The Psychedelic Explorer's Guide: Safe, Therapeutic, and Sacred Journeys* (Rochester, VT: Park Street Press, 2011).

- The "two days a week" protocol, which is similar to the previous one but sets the intake on two specific, nonconsecutive days of the week (for example, Monday and Thursday).
- The "alternate day" protocol, which proposes taking a microdose every other day (for example Monday, Wednesday, and Friday).
- The Stamets protocol, which consists of consuming a combination of a microdose of psilocybin with Lion's Mane mushroom and niacin (vitamin B3) for four days, and then resting for three days, taking only Lion's Mane.

To date, there have been mixed results in the clinical trials designed to evaluate this practice. While most studies to date have shown that people who believe they are microdosing improve in some areas, they have not been able to strongly demonstrate that microdosing is better than placebo. There was one study that found small differences but attributed them to the design of the study itself,[23] so it is possible that said improvement effect could be the result of autosuggestion, and a recent review found some modest improvements in neural connectivity and social cognition, as well as mood and perception of pain and time.[24] Still, it is a field in which much remains to be investigated.

What has been observed is that small doses of LSD, even in this microdose range, produce BDNF release in humans,[25] which might potentially be very interesting for neuroplasticity and even for neurogenesis, although this release is not something exclusive to psychedelic substances.

Unfortunately, trying it for long periods of time is not risk-free, as

---

23. Szigeti et al., "Self-Blinding Citizen Science to Explore Psychedelic Microdosing," *eLife* 10 (March 2021): e62878.

24. Robin J. Murphy, Suresh Muthukumaraswamy, and Harriet de Wit, "Microdosing Psychedelics: Current Evidence From Controlled Studies," *Biological Psychiatry: Cognitive Neuroscience and Neuroimaging* 9, no 5. (May 2024): 500–511.

25. Nadia R. P. W. Hutten et al., "Low Doses of LSD Acutely Increase BDNF Blood Plasma Levels in Healthy Volunteers," *ACS Pharmacology & Translational Science* 4, no. 2 (April 2021): 461–66.

there are (at least in theory) potential risks[26] for the heart when consuming psychedelics on a daily basis. Although it is true that at such low doses it is not known whether they can represent a real danger or not, some researchers have already warned that it might be possible.

OTHER LINES OF RESEARCH FOR POSSIBLE FUTURE APPLICATIONS

There are plenty of potential new lines of research involving psychedelics that are starting every year and there are many to come, but it takes time for the scientific process to start producing enough evidence and publications to consolidate or discard those new lines of research. Just to give an idea to the reader, here are some other lines of research currently in process for the possible future application of psychedelics:

- Creativity and problem solving
- Learning disorders
- Obsessive-compulsive disorder
- Language disorders such as stuttering or dyslexia
- Social anxiety in people with autism
- Anorexia
- Tinnitus
- Phobias
- Palliative care
- Chronic pain
- Grief

---

26. See note 25 (Hutten et al.); Joshua D. Hutcheson et al., "Serotonin Receptors and Heart Valve Disease—It Was Meant 2B," *Pharmacology & Therapeutics* 132, no. 2 (November 2011): 146–57. See also Antonin Rouaud, Abigail E. Calder, and Gregor Hasler, "Microdosing Psychedelics and the Risk of Cardiac Fibrosis and Valvulopathy: Comparison to Known Cardiotoxins" *Journal of Psychopharmacology* 38, no 3 (January 2024); 217–224.

7

The Applications, Effects, Dosages, and Risks of Different Psychedelic Substances

PSILOCYBIN ("MAGIC MUSHROOMS")

Definition, Composition, and Origin

Psilocybin (also called 4-PO-DMT or 4-phosphoryloxy-N,N-dimethyl-tryptamine), formerly marketed as Indocybin by Sandoz in the 1960s, is a naturally occurring psychedelic substance from the tryptamine chemical family (they have similarities to serotonin). It is found in up to 180 varieties of fungi, distributed throughout all continents, but especially in tropical and subtropical forests. The most common and popular species of psilocybin mushrooms are: *Psilocybe cubensis, Psilocybe subcubensis* and *Psilocybe semilanceata*, commonly known as "magic mushrooms" or "liberty caps." A recent study dates the production of the psilocybin molecule in psilocybe mushrooms as starting between ten and forty million years ago.

Although these mushrooms usually also contain other active ingredients, such as psilocin (4-HO-DMT) and baeocystin (4-HO-NMT), psilocybin is considered their main active ingredient, since it is the one with the greatest presence and chemical stability, which makes it the

Psilocybin molecule.

most abundant substance in mushrooms when consumed. Paradoxically, it is not the psilocybin that ultimately acts on the brain. When it enters the body, it is converted into psilocin, and it is this psilocin that is responsible for most of the final psychedelic effects.

Applications

Throughout history, psilocybin mushrooms have had various religious, ritual, and shamanistic uses; in fact, there are prehistoric artistic representations on practically every continent. In the Aztec language, these mushrooms were called *Teonanacatl*, or "meat of the gods."

Currently, its use may be associated with recreation, with self-exploration, self-knowledge, personal development, and spirituality, and therapeutically it is being investigated for the treatment of conditions such as depression, anxiety, post-traumatic stress disorder, addictions, and obsessive-compulsive disorder, making it the most studied psychedelic substance today, along with MDMA and ketamine.

Like other tryptamines, it has also been successfully used for the treatment of cluster headaches.

Forms and Routes of Administration

Psilocybin is commonly ingested orally as a component of a mushroom or truffle, both of which can be found fresh or dried. These mushrooms and truffles can be purchased from a drug supplier or grown at home with one of the many home grow kits available today. They can also be found in the field, but given the huge variety of similar mushrooms in nature,

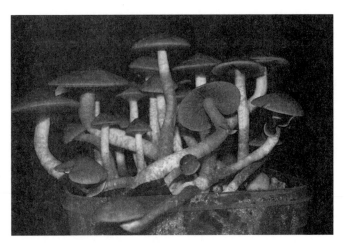

Psilocybe cubensis
"golden teacher"
mushrooms.
Photo by Mädi.
(See also color
plate 14.)

many of them poisonous, this practice can be very risky for amateurs. The consumption of psilocybin orally is done by chewing the dried or fresh mushrooms, or by preparing a tea with water, or by preparing a drink with lemon called "lemon tek."[1] The latter method has some advantages, such as reducing the nausea usually experienced when eating raw mushrooms, improving absorption, and speeding up the onset of effects.

In clinical research, psilocybin is often used in pure form that can be obtained by isolating the molecule from the mushroom or by synthesizing the molecule in a lab. The latter process it typically used to obtain a GMP (good manufacturing practices) final product, for pharmaceutical standards. It is usually administered orally isolated in capsules, but has also been administered intravenously, especially in neuroimaging studies, to speed up its effects and see the changes in brain activity.

Pharmacology and Effects

After mushrooms or truffles are ingested, eaten raw or in tea form, psilocybin is absorbed by the stomach, enters the blood, and begins to convert to psilocin within the body through a process called dephosphorylation. This psilocin, which is responsible for the psychoactive effects, reaches the brain and activates the 5-HT2a serotonin neuroreceptors (like most psychedelic substances) and the 5-HT1a receptors in the neurons of the

---

1. Preparation of squeezed lemon juice with crushed or powdered mushrooms that, after soaking for a few minutes, is strained and drunk.

brain, triggering the psychedelic effects that we have described in previous chapters.

The physical effects of psilocybin are few, mainly dilation of the pupils and a slight increase in heart rate and blood pressure, especially in high doses and in direct relation to the psychological effects the person is experiencing.

The psychological effects of psilocybin are numerous and highly dependent on variables like dose, person, and context. The most characteristic are major changes in sensory perceptions, cognition, emotions, and consciousness.

Changes in sensory perceptions can manifest visually, with color enhancement, distortions in the shapes and movements of things, and colorful kaleidoscopic visions with closed eyes. Synesthesia and increased tactile, thermal, and tingling sensations may appear. Hearing disturbances can lead to an increased appreciation of music and sounds.

Cognitive alterations can be perceived as positive and pleasant or negative and difficult, and it is common for psychedelic experiences to include good stages and more difficult moments, which is why they are called trips.

They commonly bring up biographical and personal content, like relationships with significant people in your life or other personally meaningful content. In high doses and controlled contexts, psilocybin can induce mystical experiences, with the dissolution of personal and ego boundaries, and oceanic feelings, which can be experienced with great peace and transcendence, but can also generate anxiety and even fear.

Psilocybin can reduce the activity of the amygdala, the center of the brain related to fear, and therefore induce a positive bias in the perception of ourselves and our environment. It can also produce a lot of laughter.

It also tends to produce a feeling of physical tiredness that is less conducive to movement or exploration than other psychedelics such as LSD.

Dosage

Mushrooms, when dried, lose about 90% of their weight, which was in the form of water, so, in general terms, each gram of dried mushroom is equivalent to 10 g of fresh mushroom.

Although some psychoactive substances are dosed taking into account the weight of the person receiving the substance, in the case of psilocybin this does not seem to have much influence on the final effect, which is why fixed doses are typically used.[2]

The dose of pure psilocybin used in research is around 20–25 mg, which would be equivalent to about 2.5–3 g of dried psilocybe mushrooms (about 20 or 25 g of fresh psilocybe mushrooms), if we consider the contribution of the small amounts of psilocin that accompany it, especially if they are fresh.

Those who consume it in microdoses look for a tenth of the active dose, equivalent to about 2 mg of psilocybin or 250–300 mg of dried psilocybe mushroom, but for some people that might be too much and they may prefer even smaller doses to avoid feeling the slight effects.

The concentration of psilocybin in a mushroom or truffle will depend on many factors, such as its species, its exposure to light, its growth and harvest time, its level of drying, the specific part of the mushroom, its age, and its conservation (psilocybin, like other compounds, tends to degrade over time after harvesting and drying). Therefore, it is very difficult to know the concentration of psilocybin, psilocin, and baeocystin in a sample of mushrooms without doing a chemical analysis of it, but some approximate average concentrations per species collected in the literature[3] are:

Species	% Psilocybin by Weight of Dried Mushroom
Psilocybe azurescens	1.78%
Psilocybe semilanceata	0.98%
Psilocybe cubensis	0.63%
Psilocybe cyanescens	0.85%
Psilocybe tampanensis (truffles)	0.68%
Panaeolus cyanescens/Copelandia cyanescens	2.51%

2. Albert Garcia-Romeu et al., "Optimal Dosing for Psilocybin Pharmacotherapy: Considering Weight-Adjusted and Fixed Dosing Approaches," *Journal of Psychopharmacology* 35, no. 4 (April 2021): 353–61.
3. Paul Stamets, *Psilocybin Mushrooms of the World: An Identification Guide* (New York: Random House Digital, 1996).

As for the doses, various levels can be established depending on the intention of consumption: microdoses (below the threshold of the minimum psychoactive dose) for those seeking imperceptible effects, low doses or medium doses for a first approach to the substance or recreational use, and high doses for therapeutic work or mystical experiences.

Doses	Dried Psilocybe Cubensis Mushrooms: Oral	Pure Psilocybin: Oral
Microdose	< 0.25 g	< 2.5 mg
Minimal Psychoactive	0.25–0.5 g	3–6 mg
Low	0.5–1 g	6–10 mg
Medium	1–2.5 g	10–20 mg
High	2.5–5 g	20–35 mg
Very High (higher risks)	> 5 g	> 35 mg

Duration

The following table shows some approximate times for both the total duration of the experience and the duration of the different phases. The absorption/latency phase is the time that passes from when the substance is ingested until its effects begin to be noticed. The rise phase (or come-up) is the time between starting to feel the initial psychedelic effects until their maximum intensity is reached. The plateau phase (or peak) is the time of maximum stable psychoactive effects of the substance, in which the majority of the psychedelic experience takes place. The descent phase (or come-down) is the time starting when these effects fade until they become insignificant, and the brain activity gradually returns to normal. The residual phase or afterglow refers to the time in which psychological normality has already returned, but there are still some slight sensations present in the background, usually positive.

Duration of Effects	Psilocybin: Oral
Total Duration	4–7 hours
Absorption/Latency	15–60 minutes
Rise	15–30 minutes
Plateau	2–4 hours

Duration of Effects	Psilocybin: Oral (Cont'd)
Descent	1–3 hours
Residual/"Afterglow"	6–12 hours

Specific Risks

Like other classic psychedelics, psilocybin has a very low level of toxicity and no addictive potential. However, it presents risks on a psychological level, especially in people with latent psychiatric disorders or a propensity for them.

All psychedelics can produce feelings of dizziness or nausea at the onset of their effects, but psilocybin mushrooms can be especially prone to this, especially if eaten raw (and not in tea form) and on a full stomach. In addition, a full stomach can also greatly attenuate the desired effects of psilocybin, which is why it is usually consumed when fasting for at least 4–6 hours. To reduce nausea and speed absorption, some people prepare lemon tek. Combining psilocybin with other drugs and medications, especially tramadol and lithium, can increase the risk of having a seizure or even serotonin syndrome.[4] There is also a risk of using the wrong mushroom or consuming others that may be toxic, especially if they are collected in the wild.

Despite a well prepared set and setting, sometimes you could encounter difficult experiences (commonly called bad trips) when you may feel anxiety, fear, paranoia, confusion, agitation, space–time disorientation, or a feeling of "going crazy" or dying. But they are usually transient and rarely last beyond the pharmacological effect of the substance. Eating small amounts of light food may help reduce these effects. There are also strategies described in the section called Managing "Bad Trips" and other Psychedelic Emergencies, in the chapter Psychedelic Risks and Harm Reduction Strategies of this book, that can help.

At the psychiatric level, the consumption of psilocybin by people with a propensity for psychosis, bipolarity, or schizophrenia, or a family

---

4. A potentially life-threatening condition resulting from an excess of serotonin in the brain, typically caused by drug interactions or overdose and characterized by symptoms such as confusion, fever, shivering, sweating, rapid heart rate, and muscle stiffness.

history of any of these, can increase the risk of triggering episodes. In very rare cases it can cause flashbacks or hallucinogen persisting perception disorder (HPPD), but this phenomenon is still very under-researched.

LSD ("ACID")

Definition, Composition, and Origin
LSD (German initials for Lysergic Acid Diethylamide), known on the street as "acid" or "blotter," formerly marketed as Delysid by Sandoz in the 1950s and 1960s, is a semi-synthetic drug with psychedelic effects from the chemical family of tryptamines (they have similarities with serotonin). They are derived from lysergic acid and are present in various plant and fungal species, such as the well-known ergot (*Claviceps purpurea*).

Applications
LSD began to be used as a psychotomimetic (a substance that apparently mimics psychosis), but it was soon discovered that it had great therapeutic potential to help people with alcoholism overcome their addiction, and terminal cancer patients lose their fear of death and come to terms with their life.

Also, like other tryptamines, it has been used successfully in the treatment of cluster headaches.

Since its prohibition at the end of the 1960s, its use has been eminently recreational, for personal development, or in *underground*

LSD molecule.

therapy. Now, it is being investigated again clinically for the treatment of various psychological disorders such as depression, anxiety, and various addictions. Although given its long duration of effects and less tendency to induce introspection, it has less clinical interest compared to psilocybin.

Forms and Routes of Administration

LSD is a salt, but its active doses are so minimal (in the order of micrograms, that is, millionths of a gram) that they are almost invisible to the human eye and, therefore, dosage using a scale is very difficult. For this reason, it is normally dosed by diluting it in water or another solvent, such as ethyl alcohol, and administering that solution directly orally in the form of drops; or placed on a blotting paper (or any other porous, transportable material), and allowed to dry, leaving the dose of LSD "trapped" inside and ready to be transported or consumed. It is usually sold in thick blotting papers pre-cut into small squares, and with elaborate designs known as blotters or sheets.

Many people collect these beautifully designed blotters, usually empty, but also sometimes laced with LSD.

LSD is usually taken orally, although researchers have also used it intravenously. There is a myth that it is consumed applied directly to the eye, but it is, frankly, unlikely that this practice will go beyond the anecdotal.

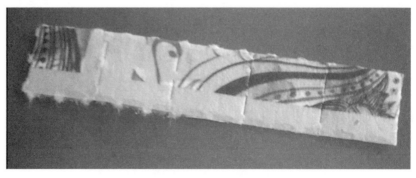

LSD blotter with five doses. Photo by Motorbase.
(See also color plate 15.)

Pharmacology and Effects

LSD reaches the blood through the digestive system and gains access to the brain. Once there, it binds to several serotonergic receptors, in particular the serotonin 5-HT2a receptor, considered to be the main one responsible for its psychedelic effects. It also binds to other receptors such as 5-HT1a, 5-HT2b, 5-HT2c, and 5-HT6, but its effects are less well understood.

Unlike other serotonergic psychedelics, LSD has some effect on dopamine and norepinephrine receptors, with a small contribution to the psychedelic experience that may be somewhat more uplifting and energetic than that induced by psilocybin.

The physical effects of LSD are few, mainly dilation of the pupils and a slight increase in heart rate and blood pressure, especially in high doses.

As in other psychedelic substances, the psychological effects of LSD are numerous and highly dependent on the variables of dose, person, and context. The most characteristic are significant changes in sensory perceptions, cognition, emotion, and consciousness.

Desired effects of this substance include (but are not limited to): euphoria, laughter, sense of perception, enlightenment, synesthesia, new ways of thinking about oneself and others, deep feelings of love and well-being, changes in the perception of time and space, spiritual experiences, and visual hallucinations (but generally distinguishable from reality).

Changes in sensory perceptions can manifest visually, with color enhancement, distortions in the shapes and movements of things, and colorful kaleidoscopic visions with closed eyes. Synesthesia and increased tactile, thermal, and tingling sensations may appear. Hearing disturbances can lead to an increased appreciation of music and sounds.

Cognitive alterations can be perceived as positive and pleasant or negative and difficult, and it is common for psychedelic experiences to include good stages and more difficult moments, which is why they are called trips.

It commonly brings up biographical and personal content, like relationships with significant people in your life or other personally meaningful content. In high doses and controlled contexts, LSD can induce mystical experiences, with the dissolution of personal limits and the ego, with oceanic feelings, which can be experienced with great peace and transcendence, but can also generate anxiety and even fear.

Compared to psilocybin, it is considered a more energetic, outgoing, and highly visual experience.

Dosage

LSD is such a powerful molecule that the active dose is almost invisible to the naked eye, so proper dilution is the only way to dose it with less risk of error. On the other hand, when it is sold already dosed in blotters, chemical analysis is the only way to know the potency and purity of a given batch.

On the market, blotters can contain a wide variety of dosages, but they are usually between 80 and 150 micrograms, which would be an average dose very common in recreational or experimental contexts of use.

Sex, body weight, sensitivity to psychedelics, and previous tolerance are factors that would determine the final potency of the effects.

Doses	LSD: Oral
Microdose	< 12 micrograms
Minimal Psychoactive	15–25 micrograms
Low	25–75 micrograms
Medium	75–150 micrograms
High	150–250 micrograms
Very high (higher risks)	> 250 micrograms

Duration

The effects of LSD are very long-lasting, ranging between 8 and 12 hours, but can reach 16 hours in very high doses. In any case, an experience never has the same intensity throughout, and it is considered that most of its effects are concentrated in the first 4–6 hours after ingestion.

Duration	LSD: Oral
Total Duration	8–12 hours
Absorption/Latency	15–30 minutes
Rise	45–90 minutes
Plateau	3–5 hours
Descent	3–5 hours
Residual/"Afterglow"	12–48 hours

Specific Risks

Like other classic psychedelics, LSD has a very low level of toxicity and no addictive potential, with documented cases of involuntary ingestion of very high doses without physiological risks or consequences. However, it presents risks on a psychological level, especially in people with psychiatric disorders or a propensity for developing them.

Like other tryptamines, LSD does not have much interaction with the cardiovascular or respiratory systems, or others. It dilates the pupils (mydriasis), and, at high doses, it can slightly raise heart pressure, heart rate, and body temperature, but it does not generally do so in a magnitude of risk, except in cases of people with previous hypertensive disease. Combining LSD with other drugs and medications, especially tramadol and lithium, can increase the risk of having a seizure or even serotonin syndrome.

Despite a well prepared set and setting, sometimes you could encounter difficult experiences (bad trips) when you may feel anxiety, fear, paranoia, confusion, agitation, space–time disorientation, or a feeling of dying or "going crazy." But the feelings are usually transient and rarely last beyond the pharmacological effect of the substance. In any case, there are also strategies described in the section called Managing "Bad Trips" and other Psychedelic Emergencies in this book that can help.

At the psychiatric level, the consumption of LSD by people with a propensity for psychosis, bipolarity, or schizophrenia, or a family history of any of these, can increase the risk of triggering episodes. In very rare cases it can cause flashbacks or hallucinogen persisting perception disorder (HPPD).

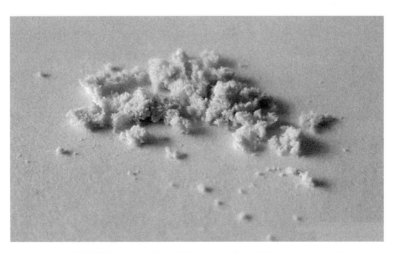

DMT molecule.

DMT/AYAHUASCA

Definition, Composition, and Origin

DMT (abbreviation for N,N-DiMethylTryptamine, also called the "spirit molecule") is a psychedelic tryptamine, from the chemical family of tryptamines (it has similarities to serotonin), and of natural origin. It can be found in a wide variety of plants (such as acacias, mimosas, and chacruna [*Psychotria viridis*]) and even in small amounts in the mammalian brain.[5]

Extraction of DMT in crystallized form, extracted from a vegetal source. Photo by DM Trott. (See also color plate 16.)

5. Jon G. Dean et al., "Biosynthesis and Extracellular Concentrations of N,N-Dimethyltryptamine (DMT) in Mammalian Brain," *Scientific Reports* 9 (June 2019): 9333.

Applications

Although the physiological role of endogenous DMT is unknown, DMT has been used for centuries as one of the main psychoactive ingredients in ayahuasca for ritualistic, religious, and therapeutic use.

Although in Western countries the use of DMT has been associated with recreational contexts (especially in the form of pure DMT crystals that are vaporized), currently, the ritual, spiritual, personal development, and therapeutic use of this Amazonian potion is also experiencing great growth and popularity in Western countries. The use of this drink in recreational or nonceremonial contexts is possible but practically nonexistent at the moment.

Likewise, research on its therapeutic potential is booming, with studies of its use, both in the form of oral ayahuasca and intravenous injection of pure DMT, for the treatment of depression, anxiety, or addictions and for its potential for neurogenesis and neuroplasticity.

Forms and Routes of Administration

DMT is usually found isolated in the form of crystallized salts that are extracted through a process of dissolution and filtration from the dried and pulverized bark of plants such as the *Mimosa hostilis*. These salts are vaporized in a glass pipe or electronic vaporizer and inhaled, the psychedelic effects are very intense and take a few seconds to appear.

DMT is also found as one of the two main active ingredients that make up the sacred Amazonian drink ayahuasca, or "yage," known as "medicine" in traditional consumption contexts. This drink also contains substances that allow DMT to be active orally because, otherwise, the human body contains enzymes called monoamine oxidases that destroy DMT if it were ingested alone. These substances, called beta-carbolines, come from yagé (*Banisteriopsis caapi*) and act as monoamine oxidase inhibitors (MAOIs), canceling these enzymes and allowing DMT to reach the brain and exert its pharmacological psychedelic effect.

Inspired by the combination of DMT with MAOIs for oral consumption, other westernized versions of Amazonian ayahuasca have appeared, such as "mimosahuasca," which combines the DMT of

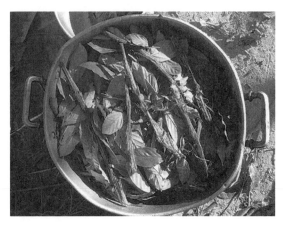

Ayahuasca ingredients before being cooked. Photo by Awkipuma. (See also color plate 17.)

a mimosa with the MAOIs present in the Mediterranean harmala (*Peganum harmala*), or the "farmahuasca," which combines DMT with MAOIs for pharmaceutical use.[6]

There is also a smokeable vegetable preparation known as "changa" that combines DMT with MAOIs on herbs in such a way that it makes it easier to smoke and prolongs the effects of DMT compared to it being vaporized alone, but it is quite exotic and not very easy to find.

Pharmacology and Effects

Whether vaporized or taken orally accompanied by MAOIs, DMT reaches the blood and crosses the blood–brain barrier to reach the brain, where it exerts its pharmacological action by binding to the 5-HT2a serotonin neuroreceptor, as well as to 5-HT1a and 5- HT2c.

There has been much speculation about whether the DMT produced by our body has a specific function, with theories relating it to dreams, neuroplasticity, psychological change, or near-death experiences, but there are still few certainties.

Psychedelic experiences with vaporized DMT are extremely fast and intense, and very visual. The person is immersed in a trance during

---

6. Although MAOIs were used as a treatment for tuberculosis, they later began to be used as the first known antidepressants, and today they continue to exist in the pharmacopoeia and are still commercialized.

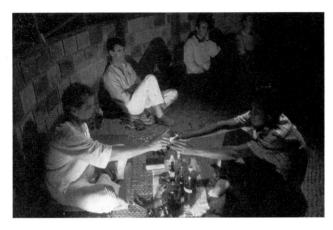

Ayahuasca ceremony at the Takiwasi center, Peru. Photo by Jaime Torres/ Archivo Centro Takiwasi.

which they lie down with their eyes closed and without much interaction with the environment.

The experience combines intense kaleidoscopic images, to the point of feeling as if they are astral travelling through galaxies, encountering other entities, which can manifest in various forms and appearances. A good example of these images are the paintings and designs of the artist Alex Grey.

Instead, oral ayahuasca experiences are more similar to those that psilocybin can induce, except for a greater tendency to nausea and differences in phenomenology, intensity, and duration of effects. The ceremonial context in which the consumption of ayahuasca is carried out also endows the experience with a special imagery and meaning.

Dosage

Without a chemical analysis of the sample, the dosage of ayahuasca is very complicated to predict, because it is not a "standardized" preparation—there are many different preparations, with different concentrations of DMT, and its potency is also greatly influenced by its concentration of MAOIs.

On the other hand, if it is pure vaporized DMT, its dosage is easier to establish. Nevertheless, it will also depend a lot on the efficiency of the vaporization process, in which, depending on the temperature applied, the molecule may not be able to vaporize at all or it could burn and lose its psychoactive effects.

Doses	DMT: Vaporized
Minimal Psychoactive	2 mg
Low	10 mg
Medium	20 mg
High	40 mg
Very high (higher risks)	> 60 mg

There are many plants that contain DMT. Below is a list of some of them and their concentrations of DMT:

Plant DMT Content	% DMT in Dry Weight
Jurem (*Mimosa hostilis*)	1.7% in root bark
Chacruna (*Psychotria viridis*)	0.1% to 0.6% in leaves
Yopo (*Anadenanthera spp.*)	0.16% DMT in the pods, along with 7.4% bufotenine and 0.04% 5-MeO-DMT
Giant reed (*Arundo donax*)	0.0057% DMT along with 0.0023% 5-MeO-MMT, 0.026% bufotenine and 5-MeO-NMT
Bundleflower (*Desmanthus illinoensis*)	0.34% DMT in the root bark
Chagropanga (*Diplopterys cabrerana*)	1.3% DMT, and trace amounts of 5-MeO-DMT, bufotenine, and methyltryptamine
Harding grass (*Phalaris aquatica*)	0.1% DMT, 0.2% 5-MeO-DMT, and 0.005% bufotenine
Reed canary grass (*Phalaris arundinacea*)	0.12% DMT
Phalaris tuberosa	0.02% DMT
Salparni (*Desmodium gangeticum*)	0.057% DMT in root and leaves

Duration

There are marked differences between the duration of effects of vaporized DMT compared to the oral route in the form of ayahuasca.

Durations	DMT: Vaporized	Ayahuasca: Oral
Total Duration	5–20 minutes	4–6 hours
Absorption/Latency	20–40 seconds	20–60 minutes
Rise	1–3 minutes	30–45 minutes

Durations	DMT: Vaporized	Ayahuasca: Oral (Cont'd)
Plateau	2–8 minutes	1–2 hours
Descent	1–6 minutes	1–2 hours
Residual/"Afterglow"	10–60 minutes	1–8 hours

Specific Risks

In addition to the typical psychological risks of psychedelic substances that arise, fundamentally, from the context in which they are consumed and from the psycho-emotional state of the person who consumes them, ayahuasca tends to produce nausea and vomiting. It also presents additional physiological risks related, especially, to its content of monoamine oxidase inhibitors (MAOIs), since these substances can cause sweating, palpitation, tremors, tachycardia, and serious symptoms such as hypertensive crises and hyperpyrexia (high fever).

This presence of MAOIs also makes it very dangerous to consume ayahuasca if you are using other medications, especially antidepressants or other psychoactive drugs, like ADHD stimulants or lithium, which in combination with ayahuasca could lead to seizure and serotonin syndrome, or if you combine ayahuasca with foods rich in tyramine such as mature cheeses, nuts, chicken liver, or fish (like herring and sardines), which can cause hypertensive crises. This is another reason why people who are going to take it undergo a special diet before and after, because the pharmacological effects of MAOIs are not limited to the ayahuasca experience and could last for several days after.

Despite a well prepared set and setting, sometimes you could encounter difficult experiences (bad trips) where you may feel anxiety, fear, paranoia, confusion, agitation, space–time disorientation, or a feeling of "going crazy." But they are usually transient and rarely last beyond the pharmacological effect of the substance. In any case, there are also strategies described in the section called Managing "Bad Trips" and other Psychedelic Emergencies in this book that can help.

Although very rare, some deaths related to the consumption of ayahuasca have been reported, especially in people mixing it with other drugs and medications or suffering from previous heart conditions.

Aside from the risk of falls (and pipe burns), which makes

consumption sitting or lying down safer, experiences with DMT can be so intense that they could be unpleasant for some people.

At the psychiatric level, the consumption of DMT or ayahuasca by people with a propensity for psychosis, bipolarity, or schizophrenia, or a family history of any of these, can increase the risk of triggering episodes. In very rare cases it can cause flashbacks or hallucinogen persisting perception disorder (HPPD).

5-MEO-DMT ("TOAD")

Definition, Composition, and Origin

5-MeO-DMT (abbreviation for 5-methoxy-N,N-dimethyltryptamine, also called the "God Molecule") is a psychedelic molecule, from the chemical family of tryptamines (they have similarities to serotonin), and of natural origin. It is found in some plants (such as *Anadenanthera peregrina*, "Yopo") and, along with bufotenine [bufotenin] (5-HO-DMT) and other molecules, in the glandular secretions of at least one species of toad, the *Bufo alvarius* (*Incilius alvarius*), which inhabits the Sonoran Desert region in Mexico.

Applications

Although 5-MeO-DMT was less popular than other psychedelics, the use of plants and toads containing it has been mostly ceremonial, spiritual, therapeutic, and religious; the plants have been used for longer, while the use of the toad, *Bufo alvarius*, is much more recent. This psychedelic has become very popular lately, given its potency and its legal

5-MeO-DMT molecule.

status in many countries where it can be also found in pure synthetic form via the internet, although it is still rare to see it outside therapeutic or spiritual contexts, for purely recreational use, while extracted DMT is much more popular for this.

At the moment, there are ongoing clinical trials and several research projects focused on the molecule's possible therapeutic uses, such as depression treatment. Some observational studies have already reported very promising improvements in symptoms of depression, PTSD, and anxiety disorders among the substance's users. 5-MeO-DMT has also been shown to stimulate brain neuroplasticity, which is encouraging for the development of clinical studies with the substance for other neurological and neurodegenerative conditions.

Forms and Routes of Administration

5-MeO-DMT can be found pure, normally of synthetic origin, or accompanied by other substances, in the case of the natural glandular secretions of the *Bufo alvarius* toad.

Given the ecological problems involved in extracting 5-MeO-DMT from toad glands and its greater potential toxicity in this format, as it contains other bufotoxins, the consumption of synthetic or isolated 5-MeO-DMT is currently considered safer and is more widespread.

As with crystallized DMT, 5-MeO-DMT is usually vaporized and inhaled, although it can also be snorted.

Pharmacology and Effects

Whether vaporized or snorted, 5-MeO-DMT reaches the blood and enters the brain, where it binds primarily to serotonin neuroreceptors 5-HT2a and 5-HT1a. In addition, it produces some inhibition of monoamine reuptake, which allows it to prolong its own action but could increase its risk profile.

As with DMT, the experience with 5-MeO-DMT is brief but very intense, more so than with DMT, to the point that this molecule is considered the most powerful of all psychedelics. It also has a longer duration than DMT.

If DMT is known as the "spirit molecule," 5-MeO-DMT is

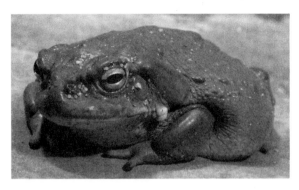

Incilius alvarius toad, also known as *Bufo alvarius*. Photo by Holger Krisp.

considered the "God molecule," although the latter term is often applied to both substances.

Dosage

The dosage will depend on the route of consumption, the doses needed being higher by snorting than by pulmonary route (vaporized).

Doses	5-MeO-DMT: Vaporized	5-MeO-DMT: Snorted
Minimal psychoactive	1–2 mg	3–5 mg
Low	2–5 mg	5–8 mg
Medium	5–10 mg	8–15 mg
High	10–20 mg	15–25 mg
Very high (higher risks)	> 20 mg	> 25 mg

Duration

There is an important difference between snorting it and taking it via pulmonary route (vaporized).

Duration of Effects	Vaporized	Snorted
Total Duration	20–40 minutes	2–3 hours
Absorption/Latency	5–60 seconds	1–10 minutes
Rise	30–60 seconds	2–5 minutes
Plateau	5–15 minutes	10–40 minutes
Descent	10–20 minutes	30–60 minutes
Residual/"Afterglow"	15–60 minutes	1–3 hours

Specific Risks

The risks of 5-MeO-DMT vary if it is derived from the isolated molecule or the secretions of the toad, since the latter contains other substances, called bufotoxins, which can make its consumption more dangerous.

In addition to the typical psychological risks of psychedelic substances, which fundamentally arise from the context in which they are used and from the psycho-emotional state of the person who uses them, the bufotoxins of 5-MeO-DMT (from toad secretions) can be cardiotoxic, and some deaths have been reported due to this form of ingestion, especially in people with heart disease or who mixed it with other psychoactive substances or drugs.

Likewise, the 5-MeO-DMT molecule itself, both isolated and in its toad secretion form, produces some inhibition of monoamine reuptake, so its combination with other psychoactive substances, such as stimulants, antidepressants, tramadol, lithium, or other psychoactive drugs, could be risky and increase the risk of seizure or even serotonin syndrome.

Aside from the risk of falls (and pipe burns), which makes consumption sitting or lying down safer, experiences with 5-MeO-DMT can be intense enough to be unpleasant.

At the psychiatric level, the consumption of 5-MeO-DMT by people with a propensity for psychosis, bipolarity, or schizophrenia, or a family history of any of these, can increase the risk of triggering episodes. In very rare cases it can cause flashbacks or hallucinogen persisting perception disorder (HPPD).

MESCALINE ("CACTUS")

Definition, Composition, and Origin

Mescaline (3,4,5-trimethoxy-beta-phenylethylamine) is a psychedelic substance of the chemical family of phenylethylamines (it has similarities with dopamine) and of natural origin (although very few psychedelics of this chemical family are of natural origin). It is found in several species of cacti, such as peyote (*Lophophora williamsii*, which also contains other psychoactives such as pellotine), San Pedro (*Echinopsis pachanoi*), the Peruvian Torch (*Echinopsis peruviana*), and other cacti. It

Mescaline molecule.

can also be found in some species of the legume family, such as *Acacia berlandieri.*

Applications

Mescaline is a substance with a long history of ceremonial use, especially in Native American cultures, and was popular in some circles before the advent of LSD; but in today's Western world it does not have much presence in clinical and recreational settings and is viewed as exotic. It is credited with nearly six thousand years of use and is considered one of the oldest psychedelic substances used by humanity.

Its therapeutic use was studied in the 1960s, along with that of LSD and psilocybin, but given its pharmacological characteristics, it did not generate a clinical interest as strong as other substances did.

Currently, unlike other classic psychedelics, there is not much research on its clinical potential, but its use is still legal for Native Americans.

Forms and Routes of Administration

Mescaline can be found in the peyote and San Pedro cacti. Peyote can be eaten directly (it has edible "buttons") or prepared as a tea or other decoction. On the other hand, the San Pedro is a tall, columnar cactus with a lower concentration of mescaline, so it is necessary to consume a larger portion, usually prepared in the form of a very bitter decoction of the outer part of its stem, called "wachuma." Both cacti can be dried, or dehydrated, and ground into a powder to make infusions.

Like most psychoactive substances, mescaline can be administered using different routes, but it is mainly ingested orally in the form of peyote or San Pedro, eaten raw, fresh or dried, or in tea form or mixed

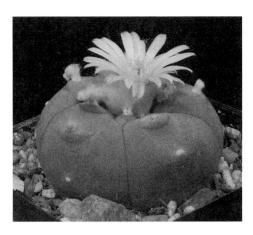

Peyote cactus in bloom,
Lophophora williamsii.
Photo by Dav Hir.
(See also color plate 18.)

in a smoothie, usually on an empty stomach to prevent nausea and maximize its absorption and effects.

The San Pedro cactus and the Peruvian Torch (a similar cactus,
also containing mescaline) are very easy to find in gardens or for sale in
nurseries, at florists, and in garden stores.

Given its long maturation period, the consumption of homegrown
peyote is even less common than that of San Pedro, although there are
grafting techniques that facilitate the accelerated growth of peyote on
the tip of a San Pedro cactus.

Mescaline can also be found isolated from the cactus, or made syn-
thetically, in the form of a salt, both as mescaline sulfate and mescaline
hydrochloride. However, it is quite an unusual substance to find and
requires large doses compared to other psychedelics. Some people buy
this salt from the dark web.

Pharmacology and Effects

Like most psychedelics, mescaline enters the blood through the digestive tract and reaches the brain, where it binds to various serotonergic
receptors, but specifically to the serotonin 5-HT2a receptor, which is
considered to be primarily responsible for its psychedelic effects. It also
binds to other receptors such as 5-HT2c, and interacts with dopaminergic receptors in a special way, due to its phenethylamine structure, different from that of other classic psychedelics such as LSD or psilocybin,
but its effects on this system are even less well known.

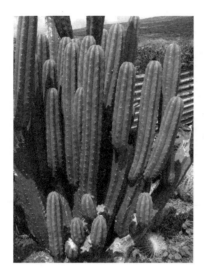

San Pedro cactus, *Echinopsis pachanoi*. Photo by Forest and Kim Starr. (See also color plate 19.)

The physical effects of mescaline are few, mainly the dilation of the pupils and the increase in heart rate and blood pressure, especially in high doses.

The psychological effects of mescaline are numerous and highly dependent on variables such as dose, person, and context. The most characteristic are significant changes in sensory perceptions, cognition, emotion, and consciousness.

Changes in sensory perceptions can manifest visually, with light and color enhancement, distortions in the shapes and movements of things, and colorful kaleidoscopic visions with eyes closed. Synesthesia and increased tactile, thermal, and tingling sensations may occur. Hearing disturbances can lead to an increased appreciation of music and sounds. There can also be a lot of laughter.

Cognitive alterations can be perceived as positive and pleasant or negative and difficult, and it is common for psychedelic experiences to include good stages and more difficult moments, which is why they are called trips.

Desired effects of this substance include (but are not limited to): euphoria, sense of perception, enlightenment, synesthesia, new ways of thinking about oneself and others, deep feelings of love and well-being, changes in the perception of time and space, spiritual experiences, and visual hallucinations (but generally distinguished from reality).

It commonly brings up biographical and personal content, including relationships with significant people in your life and other personally meaningful content. In high doses and controlled contexts, mescaline can induce mystical experiences, with the dissolution of personal limits and the ego, with oceanic feelings, which can be experienced with great peace and transcendence, but can also generate anxiety and even fear.

Mescaline is reputed to produce psychedelic experiences that are more pleasant or have fewer difficult stages than other psychedelics, and are more luminous, with oneiric[7] quality.

Dosage

Pharmacologically speaking, mescaline is not a very potent psychedelic, so doses need to be considerably large compared to others, hovering around a third of a gram (300 mg), but it is rarely taken in isolated or purified form, so amounts depend very much on the age of the peyote or how the San Pedro wachuma has been prepared. It is usually measured in number of glasses.

Cacti With Mescaline	% Mescaline: Fresh weight	% Mescaline: Dry weight
Peyote (*Lophophora williamsii*)	0.4%	3–6%
Lophophora decipiens	No data	3%
San Pedro (*Echinopsis pachanoi*)	0.12%	0.33–4%
Peruvian Torch (*Echinopsis peruviana*)	No data	0.24–0.82%
Bolivian Torch (*Echinopsis lageniformis*)	No data	0.56%
Echinopsis puquiensis	No data	0.11%–0.50%
Echinopsis cuzcoensis	No data	0.14%–0.22%
Echinopsis schoenii	No data	0.14%–0.22%

Dosages for pure mescaline or cactus mescaline typically fall within the following ranges.

7. Pertaining to dreams.

Doses	Mescaline: Oral
Microdose	< 25 mg
Minimal psychoactive	50–100 mg
Low	100–200 mg
Medium	200–400 mg
High	400–600 mg
Very high (higher risks)	> 600 mg

Duration

These times are approximate and will depend largely on the particularities of the dose, purity, person, and context.

Duration of Effects	Mescaline: Oral
Total duration	8–14 hours
Absorption/Latency	45–90 minutes
Rise	60–120 minutes
Plateau	4–6 hours
Descent	2–3 hours
Residual/"Afterglow"	6–36 hours

Specific Risks

Like other classic psychedelics, mescaline has a very low level of toxicity and no addictive potential; it could have a greater risk of elevating blood pressure than other classic psychedelics, but this risk is still low in healthy people. However, it presents risks on a psychological level, which arise fundamentally from the context of use (setting) and the psycho-emotional state of the person (set). They are especially high in people with psychiatric disorders or a propensity for them.

All psychedelics can produce sensations of dizziness or nausea at the onset of effects, but cacti with mescaline can be especially prone to it, especially if they are eaten raw (and not as a tea) and on a full stomach, which is why it is usually consumed after fasting for at least 4–6 hours. The taste of wachuma is very bitter.

Despite a well prepared set and setting, sometimes you could encounter difficult experiences (bad trips) where you may feel anxiety, fear, paranoia, confusion, agitation, space–time disorientation, or a feeling of "going crazy." But the feelings are usually transitory and rarely last beyond the pharmacological effect of the substance. Eating small amounts of light food can help reduce these effects. In any case, there are also strategies described in the section called Managing "Bad Trips" and other Psychedelic Emergencies in this book that can help.

Mixing psychedelics with other psychoactive substances increases psychological risks and can add physical risks. This is especially true for mescaline, which has more interactions, especially with stimulants, MAOIs, tramadol, lithium, and other drugs.

At the psychiatric level, the consumption of mescaline by people with a propensity for psychosis, bipolarity, or schizophrenia, or a family history of any these, can increase the risk of triggering episodes. In very rare cases it can cause flashbacks or hallucinogen persisting perception disorder (HPPD).

IBOGAINE

Definition, Composition, and Origin

Ibogaine (12-Methoxybogamine) is a substance with psychedelic and dissociative properties from the chemical family of tryptamines (they have similarities with serotonin) and is of natural origin. It is found in plants of the family *Apocynaceae* as the *Tabernanthe iboga*, *Voacanga africana*, and *Tabernaemontana undulata*. In its natural form, it is usually accompanied by other alkaloids such as ibogaline and ibogamine.

Ibogaine molecule.

Applications

It has a long history of traditional ritual and religious use in Africa, most notably in the Bwiti region, in Gabon.

Some uses of ibogaine have included the treatment of asthenia, as a stimulant, and for the treatment of depression, fatigue, and recovery from infectious diseases.

It is still a very rare substance in Western countries, where there are no known uses in the recreational field, although it is being investigated for its therapeutic uses in the treatment of addictions with very promising results. This has been an ongoing interest since the 1960s, when it was shown to have properties to treat physical and psychological addiction to opiates (for example, heroin, morphine, fentanyl, methadone).

Forms and Routes of Administration

Ibogaine is usually consumed orally, using the bark of the iboga root (*Tabernanthe iboga*), a tree that grows in West Africa, and is traditionally used in rituals and ceremonies. Ibogaine, in its natural state, is usually accompanied by other substances with psychoactive effects that add to its own, as is the case with almost all natural sources of

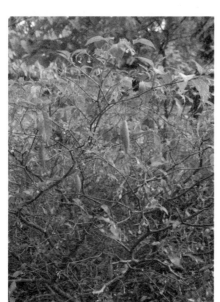

Tabernanthe iboga bush.
Photo by Marco Schmidt[1].
(See also color plate 20.)

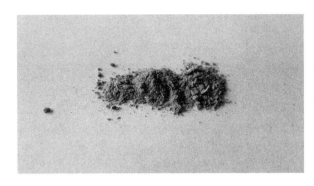

Iboga root
bark powder.
Photo by DM Trott.
(See also color
plate 21.)

psychedelics, such as mushrooms and ayahuasca. In fact, the root bark of the *Tabernanthe iboga* contains the alkaloids ibogaine, ibogaline, and ibogamine.

Pharmacology and Effects

Ibogaine is absorbed through the digestive system and reaches the blood, where it is slowly metabolized in the liver, transforming into noribogaine and other metabolites,[8] some of which may be psychoactive. Noribogaine enters the brain, where it acts on numerous receptor systems, including the dopaminergic, serotonergic (5-HT2a neuro-receptor, among others), nicotinic, GABAergic, and muscarinic systems. Some studies have found evidence that ibogaine can interrupt opioid dependence mechanisms.

Unlike most classic psychedelics, ibogaine's effects are both psychological and physical, since they also manifest in the cardiovascular system.

On a psychological level, it combines stimulating effects with psychedelic effects at high doses.

In addition to the typical psychedelic effects, it induces a longer and greater dreamlike and floating sensation, and a reevaluation of memories, past experiences, and other psychological content.

Dosage

Ibogaine typically accounts for 1% of the dry weight of the root bark of the iboga tree (*Tabernanthe iboga*).

---

8. Substances that are generated in the body's process of transformation or elimination of a substance.

Ibogaine is just an alkaloid from the iboga plant and is used almost exclusively in medical settings to treat addiction. A typical dose is 15–20 mg per kg of the person's weight, which is logically much less than when its natural unextracted version is used.

It is a substance that has not yet been studied extensively and, therefore, it is very difficult to know its exact dosage, but based on reports of use, these would be its approximate dosage levels:

Doses	Ibogaine: Oral
Minimal psychoactive	100 mg
Low	200–400 mg
Medium	400–600 mg
High	600–800 mg
Very high (higher risks)	> 800 mg

Duration

It is considered a very long-lasting natural psychedelic experience, with reports of high doses lasting for up to 24 hours or more.

Duration of Effects	Ibogaine: Oral
Total duration	8–12 hours
Absorption/Latency	45–120 minutes
Rise	60–120 minutes
Plateau	2–4 hours
Descent	4–6 hours
Residual/"Afterglow"	12–24 hours

Specific Risks

As with most psychedelics, its risks are fundamentally psychological, closely related to the variables of the context in which it is consumed (setting) and the psycho-emotional state of the person (set). However, unlike other classics such as psilocybin or LSD, ibogaine does have cardiovascular risks, since it can cause a decrease in heart rate (bradycardia) and prolong cardiac QT intervals (heart electrical wave intervals). Therefore, it should be avoided by people with a history of arrhythmias, heart attacks, heart operations, or murmurs; it is advisable to undergo an electrocardiogram and stress test before consuming it, avoiding very high doses, to reduce risks as much as possible.

It can have pharmacological interactions with foods or drugs that are metabolized by the CYP450 enzyme, so its consumption should be avoided with any other substance using this same metabolic enzyme, as it could pose additional risks.

Despite a well prepared set and setting, sometimes you could encounter difficult experiences (bad trips) where you may feel anxiety, fear, paranoia, confusion, agitation, space–time disorientation, or a feeling of "going crazy." But they are usually transitory feelings and rarely last beyond the pharmacological effect of the substance. In any case, there are also strategies described in the section called Managing "Bad Trips" and other Psychedelic Emergencies in this book that can help.

At the psychiatric level, the consumption of ibogaine by people with a propensity for psychosis, bipolarity, or schizophrenia, or a family history of any of these, can increase the risk of triggering episodes. In very rare cases it can cause flashbacks or hallucinogen persisting perception disorder (HPPD).

MDMA ("ECSTASY")

Definition, Composition, and Origin
MDMA (abbreviation for 3,4-methylenedioxymethamphetamine), better known as "ecstasy," "Molly," "X," "XTC," "E," "hug drug," or "love drug." It is a synthetic psychoactive drug with entactogenic/empathogenic, stimulant, and atypical psychedelic effects from the chemical family of phenylethylamines (which structurally resemble dopamine).

MDMA molecule.

Applications

Since its popularization in the early 1980s, MDMA has had psycho-therapeutic use (which was interrupted and forced underground by its prohibition in the mid-1980s) and recreational use, closely associated with rave culture.

It is currently a very popular recreational drug, especially in clubs, music festivals, and in the electronic music scene. But also in more intimate settings, among couples and friends.

Research into its therapeutic properties in the context of MDMA-assisted psychotherapy is very promising and growing, with a few very promising phase 3 studies for its use in PTSD treatments having been recently concluded and published, and another one to come. MDMA is getting closer to being accepted for medical use in the U.S. and Europe, while Australia already authorized its therapeutic use in treatment-resistant PTSD patients, since July 2023. There are many other potential uses currently being researched, including alcoholism, couples therapy, terminal anxiety,[9] and social anxiety in people with autism.

Forms and Routes of Administration

MDMA is usually found in two main forms: pills or crystal (known as "molly"). This crystalline form of MDMA should not be confused with "crystal meth," a much more powerful and toxic drug with pure stimulant effects and none of the empathogenic/entactogenic effects. Like most drugs, MDMA could be consumed via different routes, but it is mainly taken orally, in the form of crystal or designer pills, or inhaled in powder form.

In Europe, the purity of these crystals is lately around 80 percent MDMA by weight, making it a fairly pure substance. Outside of Europe, purity tends to be lower and may appear mixed with some psychoactive adulterants, like unscheduled new psychoactive drugs, such as cathinones.

---

9. The intense fear and emotional distress experienced by individuals who are facing the end of their life, often related to the anticipation of death and the unknown.

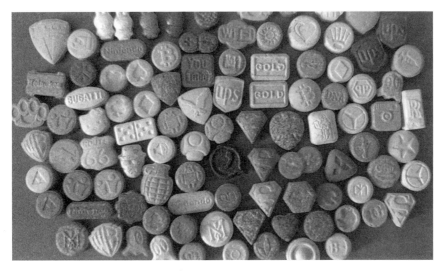

Ecstasy pills (MDMA). Photo via the Rave Jungle website.
(See also color plate 22.)

As for its presentation in the form of pills, they usually come in different colors and shapes with different logos, but with a highly variable concentration of MDMA. In recent years, their average MDMA content has increased considerably, currently exceeding 150 mg per pill in many cases and 200 mg in some, which makes it more dangerous to consume them whole and less risky to consume them in quarters or halves.

In some contexts, MDMA is snorted to accelerate its onset of effects, and even injected, like in chemsex[10] contexts sometimes, although this greatly increases its risks and changes its effect profile.

Pharmacology and Effects

Whether taken orally or snorted, MDMA reaches the blood and gains access to the brain. MDMA acts mainly as a serotonin, norepinephrine, and dopamine releasing agent in the brain, increasing their concentration in neuronal synapses. It also acts as a reuptake inhibitor of these three neurotransmitters, especially serotonin, facilitating their

---

10. Recreational practice that combines long sessions of sex with high drug use, sometimes intravenously, significantly increasing the risks that may be associated when both practices are done separately.

accumulation. It also increases the concentration of the hormonal neu-rotransmitters vasopressin and oxytocin, related to bonding, trust, or sociability.

MDMA also has weak agonist activity at serotonin 5-HT1 and 5-HT2 receptors, the latter closely related to its mild psychedelic effects, which are more noticeable at high doses but fall short compared with classic psychedelics like psilocybin or LSD, which is why it is considered a semipsychedelic or an atypical psychedelic.

At a systemic level, these effects increase the activation of the pre-frontal cortex (responsible for executive functions, among other things) and reduce the activation of the amygdala (the brain's fear response cen-ter), activating reward pathways.

All these mechanisms promote feelings of happiness, love, emotion-ality, and positivity, along with increased empathy, self-esteem, and self-acceptance. The desired effects of this substance also include euphoria, relaxation, tactile pleasure, music appreciation, sexual arousal, and energy.

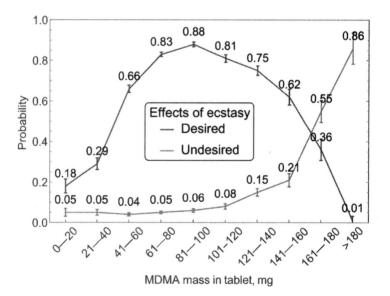

MDMA mass in tablet, mg

The dosage of MDMA that maximizes the positive effects,
without greatly increasing the risks, is around 80–100 mg.
Image from "Linking the Pharmacological Content of Ecstasy Tablets to the
Subjective Experiences of Drug Users," Brunt T. M., Koeter M. W.,
Niesink R. J., van den Brink W.

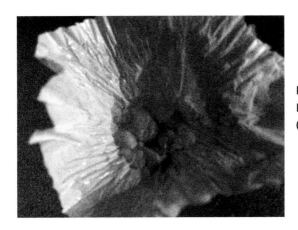

MDMA in crystals.
Photographer unknown.
(See also color plate 23.)

Dosage

There are several ways to dose crystal/powder MDMA, but the general rule of thumb is to take 1–2 mg per kilo of the person's weight, with 1 mg per kilo being a low dose, 1.5 mg per kilo a medium dose, and 2 mg per kilo a high dose. For example, the dose for a 70 kg person would range from 70 mg (low dose), 100 mg (medium dose), to 140 mg (high dose), depending on prior tolerance and the intensity of experience sought.

But, as a general rule, the doses that best balance the positive effects against the risks are in the range of 80–120 mg, with 120 mg being the usual dose used in MDMA-assisted psychotherapy in highly controlled settings.

Doses	Pure MDMA: Oral
Minimal psychoactive	25 mg
Low	25–75 mg
Medium	75–125 mg
High	125–150 mg
Very high (higher risks)	> 150 mg

If you take MDMA in pill form, due to the high dosage of modern pills (over 150 mg in many cases, and over 250 mg in some cases), it is always less risky to try a quarter and wait for the effects before deciding whether to take another quarter.

Duration

If taken orally, its effects take 30 to 60 minutes to appear (or longer, depending on stomach contents), peak in 1.5 to 2.5 hours, and last for a total of 3 to 6 hours, depending very much on the dose consumed, the body characteristics and the tolerance of the user. If snorted, those times are shortened, but the subjective effects are generally considered less positive.

Duration of Effects	MDMA: Oral
Total duration	3–6 hours
Absorption/Latency	30–60 minutes
Rise	15–30 minutes
Plateau	90–150 minutes
Descent	60–90 minutes
Residual/"Afterglow"	12–48 hours

Specific Risks

Although at moderate doses and in physically and psychologically healthy people, MDMA (ecstasy) is considered quite safe and generally produces very positive experiences, it has more risks for the body than classic psychedelics, given its stimulant profile. At high doses or in people with health problems, it can pose cardiovascular risks (such as heart attacks, strokes, arrhythmia, tachycardia, high blood pressure), dehydration, hyperthermia (even heatstroke), stimulant psychosis, hyponatremia,[11] and others that may derive from the combination with other substances.

Specifically, the risks to watch out for when consuming MDMA are:

- Dehydration: Preventable if you consume water (or isotonic drinks) on a regular basis, avoiding the consumption of other dehydrating agents such as alcohol.

---

11. Hyponatremia is a medical emergency related to a drop in sodium in the body, which occurs very rarely but could happen during MDMA consumption if a very large amount of water is consumed. It can be prevented by avoiding excessive consumption of water and drinking electrolyte drinks containing sodium.

- Hyperthermia: Due to its stimulating properties, the effects on the serotonergic system, dancing, and the increase in the metabolic rate, the body temperature could increase a lot, generating a risk of heatstroke in adverse conditions.

- Hyponatremia: Drinking too much water can affect the balance of sodium and other minerals in the body and, in large amounts, water can be toxic and even deadly if no sodium is provided.

- Hangover, "crash," or "mid-week blues:" If high and/or frequent doses are used, MDMA hangovers could present as a form of low mood, tiredness, irritability, or sadness. It usually comes on after two or three days (that is why it is called "mid-week blues"), and usually lasts no more than a day or two, but it could last longer depending on the person and dose consumed. Some people use nutritional supplements with 5-HTP (or other serotonin precursors like tryptophan) when the effects of MDMA wear off to mitigate these hangovers.

- Previous psychiatric disorders: The use of MDMA by people with a propensity for psychosis, bipolarity, or schizophrenia, or a family history of any of these, can increase the risk of triggering episodes.

Given its markedly positive effects, the risk of having a bad trip-type experience is even lower than those of classic psychedelics, although with high doses in unprepared people and in inappropriate contexts, episodes of anxiety, dizziness, confusion, disorientation, or discomfort can sometimes occur.

The long-term risks of repeated use of MDMA depend largely on the frequency and doses consumed. Frequent or high doses could cause psychological disorders, neurotoxicity, cardiovascular diseases, and even addiction. The main risks include:

- Depression: Although infrequent, the most common psychological disorder of long-term, repeated high dose MDMA abuse is depression.

- Neurotoxicity: It has long been debated whether MDMA produces relevant neurotoxicity,[12] since its consumption seems to be neuro-toxic for serotonergic neurons and induces indirect excitotoxicity[13] on mammalian brains—although the extent of this phenomenon, its clinical manifestations and long-term impact on human cognition, remains unclear. The intake of some antioxidant nutritional supplements together with ecstasy (such as alpha-lipoic acid [ALA], n-acetylcysteine [NAC], acetyl-L-carnitine [ALCAR], vitamins C and E, magnesium) seem to potentially reduce this risk of neurotoxicity, at least in some animals.

- Addiction: Although not on the same level as other pure stimulants like cocaine or methamphetamine, long-term abuse of MDMA may present some risk of psychological and physical addiction, especially in recreational use.

Due to the high purity of MDMA in recent years (mainly in Europe, the main world producer) there is a risk of overdosing, but there are also risks due to its adulteration in some markets (mainly in the American continents and Australia). So, if you are going to consume MDMA acquired on the black market, it is highly recommended to perform chemical drug testing before consumption. This can be done by a colorimetric reagent test,[14] or by contacting drug testing services for risk and harm reduction, such as those offered globally by Energy Control,[15] DrugsData[16] (formerly EcstasyData), or other local harm reduction organizations.

Mixing MDMA with other psychoactive substances increases its risks. Mixing it with other stimulants (caffeine, cocaine, amphetamines) can be problematic because it can exacerbate their stimulant properties. It can also be risky to mix it with depressants (such as GHB, benzodiaz-

---

12. Many psychoactive substances, both legal (like alcohol) and illegalized (like methamphetamine), can produce neurotoxicity, but usually at low levels if used sporadically and in moderate doses.

13. Toxicity that occurs due to the overexcitation of neurons, caused by many stimulants.

14. Sold online, especially Marquis, Mecke, and Mandelin reagents.

15. See the Energy Control International website for more information.

16. See the DrugsData website for more information.

epines, ketamine, or cannabis) as they could increase dizziness and nausea, while masking its stimulant effects, which could lead to overdosing both—with all the effects, risks, and increased amnesia associated with them. Mixing MDMA with alcohol increases its thermal and dehydration risks, as well as being unpleasant, especially at first, with dizziness and nausea, despite being a short-lived side effect.

The effects of MDMA can take a long time to kick in (up to 90 minutes or longer), especially if taken on a full stomach (not recommended), so it's risky to get impatient and, thinking it is not working, re-dose before noticing the effects of the first dose. It is a common mistake, and you may discover that you have taken too high a dose when the combined effects of several doses finally kick in, but by then it's too late to change the course.

It's important to be aware of the body temperature and stay cool, especially if dancing. Stimulants in general, but MDMA in particular, can sometimes increase body temperature to dangerous levels. To prevent this and an eventual heatstroke, it is advisable to stay well hydrated with isotonic drinks or water (without overdoing it). Avoid exposing yourself to the sun or wearing too much clothing indoors; take breaks to rest, hydrate, and refresh yourself if dancing for long hours, and check from time to time for signs of excessive body temperature. Elevated body temperature also increases the potential for excitotoxicity of stimulants.

In the case of MDMA, like other drugs, it is important to avoid using it very regularly. Potential harm increases with dose and frequency of use, and tolerance and the risk potential of addiction increase as well. In general, it is stated that to reduce the long-term risks of MDMA, it should never be taken more frequently than once a month, and ideally less often than once every three to four months. With MDMA and other psychoactive substances, less is more.

Both snorting and injecting MDMA increase the damage potential of the substance. If snorted, it is important to reduce the dose, powder the substance well to reduce damage to the nose, use a clean tube (avoiding rolled-up bills) and not share it with other people to avoid contagion of respiratory diseases or even hepatitis, and finish by cleaning the inside of the nose with saline water.

Very high blood pressure or heart rate, muscle stiffness, very high body temperature, confusion, strong hallucinations, psychosis, extreme agitation, despondency, or unconsciousness are all signs of an overdose or a potentially life-threatening reaction to the substance.

MDMA overdoses are rare, and when they do occur, it is usually moderate, but may be fatal in some cases. So, when in doubt, it is always safest to collect as much information as possible about what the person has taken and about any other health conditions they may have, and call emergency services to take care of the situation. But if this is not possible, or while they arrive, it is important to stop the person from taking any other substance, keep them in a safe, cool, calm environment, hydrate them, and cool them down if necessary.

If the person is unconscious, it is important not to give them liquids or food to avoid choking, and keep them in recovery position.[17] If they stop breathing, resuscitation (CPR) should be started. There is no specific antidote for an MDMA overdose, so the general treatment is to monitor the person while the MDMA content in the blood decreases, keeping body temperature in a safe margin or using blood pressure lowering drugs if necessary. Medical doctors can use benzodiazepines and cardiac medications to reduce the over-activation, but the use of antipsychotics on MDMA overdoses should be avoided due to the risk of heatstroke.

KETAMINE

Definition and Origin
Ketamine (also known as "Special-K," "KitKat," "K," or Ketalar) is a synthetic drug from the psychoactive class of semipsychedelic or atypical psychedelic dissociatives, and in the chemical family of arylcyclohexylamines. It is a synthetic compound that can be sold as a powder or dissolved in liquid in pharmaceutical vial form.

---

17. The recovery position, easy to see in any internet search, allows an unconscious person not to choke on their own vomit, if the situation arises.

Ketamine molecule.

Applications

Since its approval in 1970, it has been widely used as a human and veterinary anesthetic and sold under the brand name Ketalar, among others. Its recreational use also became popular in the rave scene of the 1980s.

Today, ketamine is still widely used in medicine. It is included in the World Health Organization's "Essential Medicines List," a list of the most effective and useful medicines that should be available in any modern clinic and health system. The use of ketamine as an anesthetic or analgesic is very common in veterinary medicine, as well as in human surgery and emergency medicine or with patients who are at risk from more conventional anesthesia, such as neonates or children. When used as an anesthetic or analgesic, it is usually administered together with a benzodiazepine to minimize its psychedelic effects.

Thanks to being an approved medicine, it was possible to conduct extensive research and use it as an off-label medication (approved drugs that are prescribed by healthcare providers for a non-approved condition) in various psychedelic-assisted therapy treatments. In 2019, a purification of one of ketamine's enantiomers, known as esketamine, was authorized for use in the treatment of treatment-resistant depression in the form of a nasal spray under the trade name of Spravato, becoming the first substance with psychedelic effects to be authorized for the treatment of a mental disorder. Nowadays, both esketamine and ketamine are widely used for this specific purpose with popularity among celebrities due to the great efficacy and high cost of ketamine-assisted therapy in fancy private clinics. Unfortunately, the therapeutic model commonly used to administer esketamine for depression in hospitals is

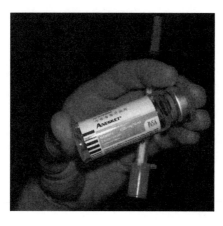

Ketamine vial, in this case for veterinary use. Photo by Psychonaught.

not a psychedelic-assisted therapy model most of the time, because most medical doctors use it relying mostly on the psychopharmacological effect of the esketamine while discarding the phenomenological value of the subjective psychedelic experience and the importance of the psychotherapy and integration.

Forms and Routes of Administration

Ketamine is often found diluted in vials of Ketalar (from Pfizer) or other brands for hospital or veterinary use, or as a bright white powder on the black market.

Like most drugs, ketamine could be consumed via different routes, but in recreational use it is mainly consumed by insufflation or orally, although in clinical settings it is most commonly injected. The new esketamine medication called Spravato is a nasal spray that is inhaled, similar to snorting it.

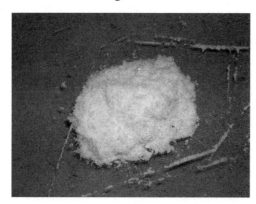

Crystallized ketamine. Photo by Coaster420. (See also color plate 24.)

Powdered ketamine for the illicit market is often obtained by drying a diluted pharmaceutical preparation, in a process that many people call "cooking," although the process is as simple as drying.

Pharmacology and Effects

Whether taken orally, through the nose, or via injection, ketamine first enters the bloodstream and then reaches the brain, where it blocks NMDA glutamate receptors (leading to loss of physical sensations, difficulty in coordination and moving, and eventually the notorious state known as "K-hole"), and acts on many other neuroreceptors at different doses. Since it does not appear to have any relevant direct action on the 5-HT2a receptor (the main psychedelic receptor), it is considered an atypical psychedelic substance.

It is a substance with a wide range of effects depending on the dose consumed, but in general terms the desired effects of this substance include (but are not limited to): dissociation, depersonalization, derealization, distortion of time and space, relaxation, insight, hallucinations, euphoria, sensation of floating, and visual distortions.

Ketamine in high doses induces psychedelic-like experiences called "falling into a K-hole" (or simply K-hole), which could be regarded in a similar way as an intense psychedelic experience, taking into account the loss of tactile sensitivity and impaired motor control, very present in the specific case of ketamine. The experience of a K-hole can be desired and pleasant for some people but very unpleasant for others.

Dosage

Unlike what happens with classic psychedelics, the dosage of this substance is very delicate since its effects can be highly variable depending on the specific dose used, making it a very important issue to take care of.

Doses	Ketamine: Snorted	Ketamine: Oral
Minimal psychoactive	5 mg	50 mg
Low	10–30 mg	50–100 mg
Medium	30–60 mg	100–200 mg
High	60–100 mg	200–300 mg
Very high (higher risks)	> 100 mg	> 300 mg

Duration

Taken orally, its effects take 10 to 30 minutes to become noticeable (depending on the contents of the stomach), with peaks reached in 45 to 90 minutes and a total duration of effects of 2 to 2.5 hours, depending very much on the dose consumed. If snorted, its effects take 5 to 10 minutes to become noticeable, peaking at 30 to 60 minutes and a total duration of effects of 1 to 1.5 hours, depending largely on the dose consumed.

Duration of Effects	Ketamine: Snorted	Ketamine: Oral
Total duration	1–1.5 hours	2–2.5 hours
Absorption/Latency	2–5 minutes	10–30 minutes
Rise	5–10 minutes	5–20 minutes
Plateau	30–60 minutes	45–90 minutes
Descent	3–6 hours	3–6 hours
Residual/"Afterglow"	2–12 hours	4–8 hours

Specific Risks

Similarly to classic psychedelics like LSD or psilocybin, ketamine has very low toxicity even at high doses and is in fact widely used in medicine at these doses. Therefore, physical and physiological safety is generally not a concern at medium doses, unless the person has accidentally taken a very high dose that could affect breathing (very, very unlikely), mixed it with other substances such as alcohol, or fainted in a swimming pool or bathtub leading to drowning. Certain activities that require coordination and reflexes such as moving about, driving, swimming, and moving things should also be avoided under its effects, as the risk of falling or having an accident increases.

Likewise, because it causes a slight increase in blood pressure (especially intracranial pressure) and subjects may undergo intense experiences that can generate anxiety, people with a history of cardiovascular disease or head injuries should proceed with special precautions or refrain from using it.

The possibility of having a difficult experience or bad trip does exist, although it can be greatly minimized with a carefully prepared set and setting. Long-lasting psychological difficulties from such an experience (negative trauma, anxiety, or long-lasting fear) are very rare, but could occur, especially if the substance is taken in high doses, for the first time, and in highly uncontrolled environments, without adequately preparing their set and setting

Although the risk of psychiatric complications is low, the use of ketamine by people with a propensity for psychosis, bipolarity, or schizophrenia, or a family history of any of these, can increase the risk of triggering episodes, especially at high doses. It can be difficult to know if someone is at risk of a psychotic reaction, especially if you are still very young, which is one of the reasons that the use of psychedelics is generally less risky in older and more mature people. In very rare cases it can cause flashbacks or hallucinogen persisting perception disorder (HPPD).

Although the long-term risks of ketamine use depend largely on the frequency of use and the doses consumed, there are some specific risks when using it frequently such as addiction,[18] urinary and bladder problems, neurotoxicity, and withdrawal syndrome. Taking it despite underlying mental conditions such as psychosis, bipolarity, or psychotic disorders could worsen the course of these disorders and contribute negatively to long-term outcomes.

The neurotoxicity of ketamine is still debated. Long-term ketamine use in humans has been linked to cognitive impairments, including deficits in memory, attention, and executive functioning. These cognitive deficits are thought to result from ketamine-induced changes in brain structure and function. However, short-term cognitive impairments seem to recover when use of ketamine is stopped. But it is always a good thing to follow the precautionary principle and avoid prolonged use or high doses.

---

18. Of the psychedelic substances, ketamine has the greatest addictive risk.

8

Psychedelic Risks and Harm Reduction Strategies

The use of drugs, whether legal (such as alcohol), controlled for medical use (such as amphetamines), or illegalized (such as ecstasy), might have applications but always carries health risks—ALWAYS. These risks can be higher or lower depending on many variables and, although the only way to completely avoid them is to not consume them, this does not mean that this is the only option, or that there aren't ways of using them with less risk if someone freely decides to take them. Therefore, there are strategies that reduce these risks as much as possible for those who are going to consume them.

Harm reduction (also called risk reduction) is an approach that accepts that, despite the laws and public health campaigns, drug use (of legal or illegalized psychoactive substances) is present in our society; instead of judging it, this approach offers a set of information, strategies, materials, practices, and tools to reduce as much as possible the risks associated with drug use for people who use them.

So far, we have mainly talked about the use of psychedelics in clinical therapeutic contexts and under professional control, but we must not forget that today the majority of people who use psychedelic drugs, or any other class (whether legal, medicinal, or illegalized), are doing it outside of the realm of clinics and laboratories.

Although they expose themselves to risks, as with any other drug-taking activity, it is not because they seek to harm their health, but rather because they obtain some benefit from their use (pleasure, fun, therapeutic benefit, self-knowledge, evasion, or socialization), and, in their opinion, these benefits are worth the risk. Although propaganda has led us to believe for years that any drug use that is not legal or medicinal is bad, science is showing that this is not always the case, and in some cases the potential benefits may indeed outweigh the risks.

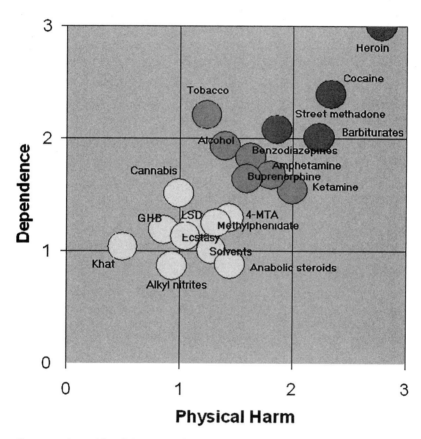

Comparative table of the risks of different substances due to their physical damage and addictiveness; most psychedelics are in the lower part of both. A rational scale to assess the harm of drugs by Apartmento2. Data sourced from the March 24, 2007, article by David Nutt, Leslie A. King, William Saulsbury, and Colin Blakemore, "Development of a Rational Scale to Assess the Harm of Drugs of Potential Misuse," *The Lancet* 369, no. 9566 (March 24, 2007): 1047–53. (See also color plate 26.)

Furthermore, putting all psychoactive substances in the same bag is a big mistake. Not only are their effects (and potential uses) very different, but their risk profiles are also quite dissimilar, even opposite, and therefore they deserve a more individualized evaluation, as we could see in the previous table on addiction and toxicity potential.

In addition, many of the dangers of the use of psychoactive substances are not intrinsic to the substance itself but are usually linked more to the lack of information about the risks and the strategies used to reduce them, and the safest context for using them. This is because many of these substances are considered a social taboo and, unfortunately, this type of information about their risks is not usually provided, as it is for pharmaceutical drugs in the form of patient information leaflets. What the evidence shows us[1] is that, if a well-informed person freely decides to consume a drug (whether legal or illegalized), and they have access to all the information and tools available to reduce those risks without necessarily giving up on the effects they seek with consumption, the person will generally apply these strategies and they will work, even though this is a field in which there is still much to be researched.

To give an example from a recreational standpoint, a person who is well-informed would not be exposed to the same risks when taking MDMA (ecstasy) at a music festival as a person who is not. The first person would take it only once a year, with trusted friends, analyzing the purity of the substance to adjust the dose and avoid toxic adulterants, consume a moderate dose according to their body weight, hydrate themselves, not mix it with alcohol or other drugs, not re-dose,[2] and would take breaks from dancing to allow their body to cool down. The uninformed person would take high doses of the substance, perform no previous analysis, mix it with alcohol and other drugs, surrounded by complete strangers, re-dose several times throughout the night, spend hours in the sun, take no breaks from dancing, and do it several times

---

1. Alison Ritter and Jacqui Cameron, "A Review of the Efficacy and Effectiveness of Harm Reduction Strategies for Alcohol, Tobacco and Illicit Drugs," *Drug and Alcohol Review* 25, no. 6 (November 2006): 611–24.
2. Re-dosing is taking a second or subsequent doses of the same substance during the same event or in a similar timeframe.

a month. Although in both cases they expose themselves to risks, there is a huge difference between the level of risk present in the first case compared to the second. Unfortunately, most uninformed recreational ecstasy users match the second profile more than the first.

There is no doubt that all drugs have risks—which is a probability of causing harm—but that does not mean that they will always cause harm, and in this sense, they can be more dangerous or less dangerous (coffee does not have the same risk as methamphetamine). However, as Paracelsus said, "the dose makes the poison," so all substances, psychoactive or not, can be harmful, and even lethal, depending on the dose, the person consuming it, and the context. Whether they finally become harmful or not will depend on a series of factors that we are now going to review in this chapter in relation to psychedelics. The damage caused

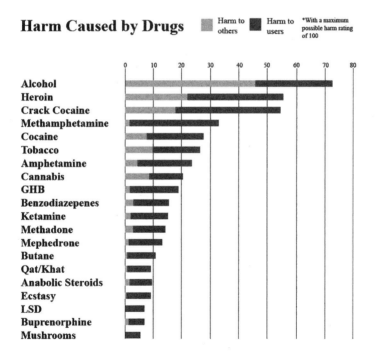

Adapted from "Drug harms in the UK: a multi-criteria decision analysis," by David Nutt, Leslie King, and Lawrence Phillips, on behalf of the Independent Scientific Committee on Drugs. *The Lancet.*

Ranking of the damage caused by the different drugs to the individual and to society in Europe. Note that ecstasy and psychedelics are at the bottom. Image from Jan van Amsterdam et al., "European Rating of Drug Harms," *Journal of Psychopharmacology* 29, no. 6 (June 2015): 655–60.

by different drugs, to individuals and to society, does not only come from the substance itself but also from the consumer and context of consumption. Note that ecstasy and classic psychedelics are usually in the lowest levels of overall harm of any psychoactive drug, legal or illegalized.

Although risk reduction is considered a part of harm reduction, they are also considered two ends of the same spectrum. Risk reduction encompasses strategies that can reduce risk and prevent harm from occurring in populations with occasional or experimental use of psychoactive substances (adequately prepared and controlled psychedelic experiences need not produce any physical or psychological harm), while harm reduction is more focused on the population with *problematic* use, where harm is already occurring, but tries to minimize it (such as syringe exchange programs among the population that regularly consumes intravenous heroin, generally with associated harm, in order to prevent the spread of infectious diseases).

There are many examples of publications,[3] tools, materials, and organizations[4] that can help with risk and harm reduction, but the main element that reduces any risk is information and knowledge. This information, to be useful, must be based on scientific evidence and not on moral dogmas or beliefs, and it must avoid judgment.

In this sense, there are strategies of enormous impact, such as knowing our state of physical and mental health, the context, learning as much as possible about a substance before consuming it (things like its doses and its risks), planning consumption in advance, chemically testing the drug for adulterants or other impurities, always starting with the minimum dose before moving on to a higher dose, not doing it on days when you are psycho-emotionally unwell, always staying adequately hydrated and nourished, not mixing it with other drugs or medications, spacing consumption over time, and, as much as possible, avoiding substances that are not chemically analyzed or that come from dealers unfamiliar to you.

---

3. Eduardo Hidalgo Downing, *Hedonismo Sostenible* [Sustainable Hedonism] (España: Ediciones Amargord, 2010).
4. Some are mentioned in the Psychedelic Resources section of this book.

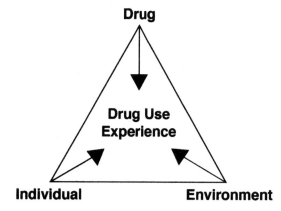

The risks and results of the consumption of a psychoactive substance can be classified into three domains: drug, individual, and environment. This model is known as "Zinberg's Triangle."

In this sense, another tool that has been shown[5] to be effective in reducing risks is drug analysis, also known as drug testing or drug checking. It is a tool that not only allows for the monitoring of drug markets from a public health perspective, but provides, together with safety advice, a way for people (who have decided to consume a drug of illegal origin) to detect if it is adulterated with substances that may be toxic. Therefore, they can decide to rule out its consumption, or adjust the dose to reduce risks if the level of purity of the drug they have acquired is not what they expected. The implementation of these information and counseling services on risk reduction and drug analysis[6] in music festivals, nightclubs, and other entertainment venues and events is a practice that has been growing for some decades in Europe, and is also increasingly widespread in North America, South America, and Australia.

Now that we have detailed the concept of risk, its multiple factors, and its variability, let's look into the main risks and reduction strategies in the use of psychedelic drugs. For this, I will divide them according to their origin into three categories: risks related to the substance (drug), to the person (set), or to the context (setting), a model known as "Zinberg's Triangle."[7]

5. Nazlee Maghsoudi et al., "Drug Checking Services for People who Use Drugs: A Systematic Review," *Addiction* 117 no. 3 (March 2022): 532–44.
6. Some of these organizations and drug testing services are mentioned in the Psychedelic Resources section of this book.
7. Norman E. Zinberg, *Drug, Set, and Setting: The Basis for Controlled Intoxicant Use,* 1986.

These three groups of variables greatly influence the risks when using any drugs. But it does not stop there, as they also influence the results of the experience itself, the effects the substance will cause (especially in the case of psychedelics), and, therefore, the result of consumption. But to be specific, let's see some examples of the variables to which I refer:

Areas of Risk	Variables
The substance (drug)	Type of drug, dose, frequency of consumption, route of administration, purity, adulterants, combinations, or interactions
Person (set)	Mental and emotional state, tolerance, allergies, illnesses, age, sensitivity, expectations, information, or preparation
Context (setting)	Environment, other people, music, lights, smell, driving, unevenness of the terrain, legal status, calendar appointments, or other responsibilities

That said, and given that the use of psychedelics outside the clinical context is a social reality today, let's see how some of the most important elements are applied to reduce their associated risks.

RISKS RELATED TO SUBSTANCE (DRUG)

Let's start by going through the most common risk sources associated with the psychoactive drug itself and how to mitigate these risks as much as possible, but not forgetting that, in the case of psychedelics in particular, variables associated with set and setting are as important or even more important.

DOSAGE, FREQUENCY OF CONSUMPTION, AND TOLERANCE

In the sixteenth century, the great alchemist Paracelsus said, "*Sola dosis facit venenum*," which translates to "Only the dose makes the poison." He continued: "All things are poison, and nothing is without poison; the dosage alone makes it so a thing is not a poison." And he was not wrong. Despite the fact that there are many decisive factors that influence the result of consuming a drug, as we have discussed, the dose is one of the most important and controllable variables, being able to determine if the desired effect will be obtained (whether therapeutic, recreational, or of a different nature), if there will be no effect at all, or if there will be an excessive effect, which would make the experience undesirable or even dangerous in some substances. An overdose, whether fatal or simply unpleasant, should be avoided at all costs.

But dosing psychoactive substances in general, and psychedelics in particular, is never an easy or risk-free task, because there are a lot of variables to consider before deciding on the exact milligrams or micrograms to use. Some of these substances are unpredictable, but most are controllable, although little known. And, because of this, it is not uncommon to see cases of people who have had problems from improper dosing that would have been easily preventable with better risk-reducing dosing information.

Although most of the classic psychedelics (psilocybin, LSD, DMT, mescaline) do not present great risks to the body in high dosages, the chances of being exposed to a psychologically difficult or extremely intense experience do increase, as do their psychiatric risks in people with predispositions.

For example, in the case of the consumption of recreational doses, if we pay attention to the safety guidelines that are usually given by risk reduction services, the optimal doses are those that maximize the pleasures (or whatever desired effect) with respect to the risks. However, as a general rule of thumb, the lower the number of re-doses and total dose consumed, the lower the risks.

Likewise, we must not forget that some of the semipsychedelic or atypical psychedelic substances explored in this book (MDMA, ibogaine, ketamine, or MAOIs from ayahuasca) can pose a risk to the body in high doses.

The doses must be adapted for the purpose of consumption and the sensitivity or tolerance of the person. It should also be noted that not all drugs are one hundred percent absorbed and reach the bloodstream. In fact, almost none are, unless administered intravenously.

Therefore, the dose is also highly dependent on the type of substance and the route of administration (oral, snorted, vaporized-inhaled, or intravenous).

In addition to bodyweight, there are other factors that must be considered when further specifying the dose. For example, it is necessary to take into account what the objective of consumption is, because a music festival is not the same as a therapeutic session. If it is the first time consuming this substance, as tolerance is nonexistent, it could feel too intense, making a lower dose generally more convenient. If you have tolerance to the substance or to other compounds of the same effects family, the dose would have to be increased a little. Consider the sex of the person—since women are generally more sensitive to the effects of certain drugs, they require lower doses. If pharmaceutical drugs (such as MAOIs, tramadol, ritonavir) or other legal (alcohol) or illegal (stimulants) drugs are being consumed, this combination would greatly increase the risks (be very careful with mixing substances). Consider the route of administration, because non-oral routes, such as snorting or smoking, require much lower doses. But, above all, there is one very important variable to consider: purity.

Before consuming any substance that comes from an illicit market, the ideal would be to have it analyzed qualitatively and quantitatively by a risk reduction analysis service, such as DrugsData or Energy Control, and thus not only prevent the presence of toxic adulterants, but also know the percentage of purity of the active compound to estimate the dosages in advance with precision. Yet, in the real world, this is not always possible, so when dosing any substance of unknown purity, it is always best to start small, with the lowest active dose, as if the purity of the substance were the highest possible. Especially if it is the first time that it is consumed or if it is from a new batch, it is better to wait and feel the effects of this testing dose before increasing the desired dose, or as the English would say, "start low and go slow"—because it is always safer to fall short than to go over. There is always the possibility of taking more, if necessary, until obtaining the desired effect. However, if you start by taking too much too quickly, there is no way to un-take it. What's done cannot be undone.

In terms of frequency of use, the less frequent the use of any psychoactive substance, the lower the risk of exposure to addiction or long-term damage. Typical psychedelics are substances that produce very intense experiences and do not encourage regular consumption (except for atypical psychedelics such as ketamine and ecstasy, which have greater potential for abuse), so their frequency of use is usually very low, normally spaced in months. Very frequent use is not a common problem.

In the case of ketamine and MDMA, it is important that their consumption is consciously spaced out over time as much as possible to minimize the risk of addiction, neurotoxicity, or psychological problems that could occur with very frequent consumption or at high doses. Likewise, another element to avoid is the development of tolerance, which would indicate that a neuroadaptation to its effects is taking place.

Tolerance is the habituation of the body or the brain to a substance that, when consumed regularly, produces an adaptation of the neurons to its effects and requires an increase in the dose to obtain the same effect, with the consequent risks that higher doses may bring. Classic psychedelics are not usually consumed regularly, but if they were, they would produce a very rapid tolerance, making their consumption on consecutive days difficult to feel, since their effects are quickly and greatly diminished, and much higher doses are required to replicate them. In fact, it usually takes about a week to completely lose tolerance after a one-off use of a classic psychedelic like LSD or psilocybin.

PURITY AND ADULTERATION

Psychedelic substances, like most illegal drugs, come from self-cultivation, underground lab synthesis, or the illicit market. In both cases there is no control over the quality of the compound, which makes it easy for dealers to adulterate the drugs, generally with the purpose of making bigger profits or defrauding the buyer with a product of lower purity that is cheaper than the one they think they are buying.

Adulteration is a fraud, attributable to the illegal status of drugs that leaves the control of the market in the hands of dealers, as opposed to the regulation of legal drugs, but it can also be dangerous to a person's health. However, not all types of adulteration are as common or dangerous as it is thought; it is convenient to make distinctions between subtypes of adulteration that occur in the market:

- Dilution or use of excipients: Using substances that, at an organoleptic level (color, texture, smell, taste), resemble the substance they intend to imitate. But they do not usually have their own relevant pharmacological effects or potential toxicity; that is, dilution is usually done with pharmacologically inert substances, such as sugars, starch, creatine,[8] and other fillers. The objective is to obtain more quantity or weight of a drug, lowering its potency, which brings in a greater profit from the sale. This type of adulteration is usually not very dangerous. An example would be the use of sugars or creatine for any drug that appears to be a white powder, such as ketamine or crushed MDMA.
- Psychoactive adulteration: The drug is mixed with other psychoactive substances (which may be legal or illegalized), the effects of which are similar and can deceive the consumer, making them believe they have purchased the intended product or that it has a higher purity than it really does. This type of adulteration is dangerous due to the health risks it may entail, since it involves a mixture of substances unknown to the consumer and modifies the psychoactive properties of the original drug. An example would be adding caffeine or cathinones to ecstasy.
- Substitution: Basically, ripping someone off. A substance is sold as if it were a drug that it actually does not contain but may have other psychoactive substances that are intended to imitate its effect. This type of fraud is one of the most dangerous since these substances may have pharmacological properties totally unknown to the user. An example would be selling 25i-NBOMe (a psychedelic with high-dose toxicity) as LSD.

---

8. A sports nutritional supplement that looks like a white powder.

• Synthesis-related impurities: The purification of a drug after synthesis is not a process that is carried out systematically in the illegal production of drugs, so many substances may contain impurities typical of the synthesis process. This adulteration can be unintentional, but very dangerous in the case of a bad synthesis that leads to toxic byproducts.

Most Common Adulterations in Psychedelic and Semipsychedelic Substances

Ecstasy/MDMA: As a result of the ban on the precursor substances[9] such as safrole and PMK used to synthesize MDMA, enforcement actions against safrole in source countries like Cambodia, some major international seizures of MDMA, and tighter controls in China's border (China was also a main precursor producer) due to the 2008 Beijing Olympic Games, there was a great international shortage of MDMA in 2008 and 2009 that greatly motivated the adulteration and substitution of MDMA worldwide. But since then, and after the discovery of new synthesis routes that made it abundant and cheap, its purity has risen a lot, especially in Europe, a main world producer, where its adulteration has been infrequent over the last decade. These are some of the adulterants that can be found sometimes in MDMA:

• Caffeine: This easily accessible, legal stimulant drug is generally used to adulterate any substance with a stimulant profile, since its stimulant effects are very noticeable to the consumer. But in high doses it can cause insomnia, tachycardia, anxiety, dehydration, and increase the risks of ecstasy.
• m-CPP: Meta-chlorophenylpiperazine has stimulant and psychedelic effects, similar to those of MDMA, but also the risk of inducing severe migraines, dizziness, vomiting, and headaches. Fortunately, it hasn't been seen as an adulterant for years.

---

9. Raw materials or chemicals used in the synthesis or manufacture of drugs, often regulated due to their potential conversion into controlled or illegal substances.

- New psychoactive substances (NPS): Various new synthetic drugs have been sold as if they were MDMA, such as cathinones (methylone, mephedrone, 3-MMC, or N,N-Dimethylpentylone) or benzofurans (such as 6-APB or 5-APB). These kinds of adulterants could be very dangerous due to the very different dosing, effects, lengths, and toxicity that they have in some cases.

Ketamine: The purity of ketamine has been relatively stable, since it commonly appears diluted with pharmacologically inert or unpurified substances, but it does not usually appear adulterated with other psychoactive substances, if at all—maybe caffeine or paracetamol on occasion. That said, it is sometimes replaced by other dissociative-type NPS that can have similar effects but pose a greater risk to those who are unaware, because they are of greater potency, duration, or intensity, or are substances that have not yet been studied, such as methoxetamine (MXE), 2-Fluorodeschloroketamine (2-FDCK), or deschloroketamine (DCK).

Psilocybin: Psilocybin is usually grown or sold in the form of psilocybin mushrooms and adulteration is very rare, but it could be substituted with other mushrooms. When these mushrooms are picked in nature, there is the risk of mistaking the mushroom species, and this could lead to taking a toxic mushroom.

LSD: LSD is not usually adulterated, but it can appear together with other products derived from its synthesis or degradation, such as iso-LSD. Sometimes there have been cases of substitution of LSD with psychedelic NPS that may be more dangerous if the user is unaware of it because they present greater risks than those of LSD or have a pharmacological profile unknown to the user. Some examples include 25i-NBOMe or DOx (DOC or DOI).

In recent years, adulterations and substitutions with fentanyl (a very dangerous opioid that should always be avoided) have appeared very rarely in some psychedelic substances in North America. It seems anecdotal or even accidental, but caution must be always given.

In a deregulated market, without controls, standards, or good information, where guile is rewarded, it is difficult to completely avoid adulteration, but there are some basic strategies that can greatly help reduce the risks of consuming an excessively adulterated product or one contaminated with toxic adulterants:

- Analyze whenever possible: There is no better way to reduce the risks of an adulterated product than to analyze it first, preferably using a service specialized in risk reduction, such as Energy Control (which, in addition to offering the service free of charge at festivals and at its locations in Spain, has an international analysis service by mail) or DrugsData in the United States. But if you don't have access to these services, there are colorimetric reagent kits on sale, testing strips for fentanyl detection, or thin-layer chromatography (TLC) for at-home testing. These kits mainly detect substitutions and some common psychoactive adulterants, although they do not quantify the purity of the substance.
- Buying from reliable and known sources: Buying a substance at a festival or nightclub from a stranger who you will never see again increases the risk of receiving an adulterated, substituted, or low-purity product, since no one will have to answer for it later.
- Do not trust appearances: If the substance does not resemble the one you seek, it may be an indication that it, in fact, isn't. However, since everything is imitable (color, smell, texture, brightness), even if it does resemble it, it is still not proof of its good quality or purity.
- Trust the effects: In this sense, one of the best risk reduction strategies is to take a small test dose to assess the effects before deciding whether to consume the "normal" dose.

ROUTES OF ADMINISTRATION

For drugs to exert their action, they have to reach the brain, and for that they have to access the bloodstream. The time it takes for a drug to reach the bloodstream to access the brain and the duration of its effects are determined by many factors, but one of the most important is its route of administration.

The greater the absorption of the route and the faster it enters the blood, the faster and more intense the effects will be. This can make the same drug more dangerous or easy to overdose (and even more addictive in some cases) depending on how it is ingested. It must also be considered that as soon as a substance enters the body, it begins to be metabolized (degraded), so the longer it takes to reach its target, the smaller the amount of the substance that will finally reach it.

Almost all psychoactive substances can be taken by almost any route, but outside of laboratories, most psychedelics are normally consumed orally or inhaled (vaporized), although some are also snorted. Here is how these methods compare:

- Oral: It is usually the slowest method because the substance has to pass through the stomach and intestine to reach the bloodstream, with a first metabolism in the liver (which can partially inactivate or release certain substances), but it is one that carries the fewest risks as long as the dose is well measured. Its speed depends a lot on the type of substance and whether the stomach is full or empty.
- Snorted: This route takes a few minutes to take effect. It reaches the blood through the nasal mucosa, but in the long run it can cause damage to the nostrils.
- Smoked/vaporized/inhaled: This method is a very quick route. It reaches the blood through the lungs and takes a few seconds to take effect, although it can cause damage to the mouth, throat, and lungs, depending on how it's done and the substance being vaporized.
- Intravenous: The fastest and most effective method, it reaches the blood directly, but carries many extra risks, such as the transmission of infectious diseases (if inappropriate hygiene measures are taken) and damage to the veins. Outside the clinical setting, it is very unusual and always inadvisable in terms of safety.

As a general rule (with several exceptions), the faster the route of administration, the lower the dose should be (because more of the substance will probably be absorbed and blood concentration will rise faster). A faster route may also usually imply the addictive potential will be greater for the same substance, although in the case of psychedelics, addiction is very rare (except in the case of ketamine, or sometimes MDMA).

MIXTURES AND COMBINATIONS

The combination of different psychoactive substances always makes their risks and manifestations more unpredictable, usually increasing their risks.

Having said this, in the real world it is unfortunately common to find the combined use of psychoactive substances, sometimes without the person being aware of it, given that we tend to forget that substances that are very commonly consumed, such as alcohol, tobacco, caffeine, cannabis, or some medications, can have a significant interaction with other psychoactive substances.

In this sense, there are psychoactive medications that can be especially dangerous when combined with other drugs, such as tramadol, monoamine oxidase inhibitors (MAOIs), lithium, opioids (used to treat pain or cough), psychostimulants (used in narcolepsy or attention-deficit/hyperactivity disorder), some anxiolytics, and some antidepressants.

Some supplements to lose weight or improve training, as well as various medicinal plants such as hypericum (St. John's wort), black cohosh, echinacea, valerian, kava, yohimbe, and ginkgo biloba may also have relevant interactions. Even some common foods such as grapefruit or certain spices can noticeably alter the metabolism of drugs and unknowingly pose a combination risk that must be taken into account.

In order to facilitate access to the scarce information available on interactions in the most common drug combinations, for some years the TripSit association[10] for risk reduction has been producing a simple chart that allows anyone to consult, in a quick and simplified way, the risks and effects of certain combinations of two drugs. This chart has evolved into a smartphone application that, without sacrificing simplicity or speed, allows access to information on a specific combination of substances. See the TripSit website for details on the drug combination chart.

On the other hand, although cannabis does not present great physiological risks when consumed alone, it can intensify or alter the effects of the other substances with which it is combined. This is mostly at the

---

10. "TripSit: Harm Reduction through Education," online.

psychological level, but also physically, and that is why mixing it with alcohol or other drugs, such as psychedelics, which some people are used to doing, does not come without risks.

RISKS RELATED TO PERSON AND CONTEXT (SET AND SETTING)

As we have seen throughout the text, most of the risks of classic or typical psychedelics are on the psychological level, and that is why the psychological variables of person and context are especially crucial to make this type of experiences carry the least possible risk.

Since psychedelics greatly amplify what we perceive happening within us and around us (even things that are already present, but we are not giving our full attention to), it is crucial that the person prop-

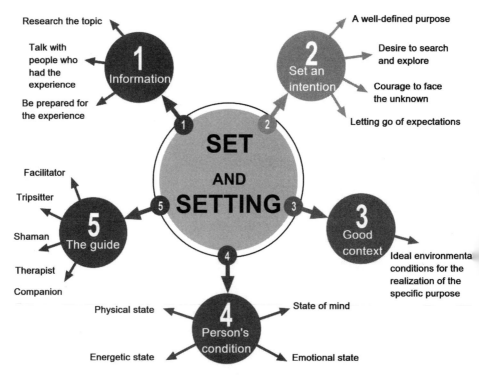

Breakdown of the different variables of set and setting that should be carefully considered to reduce the risks when using a psychedelic. Image by Jose Luis López Delgado via the Plantas Maestras website. (See also color plate 13.)

erly prepares themselves and their context to maximize the possibilities of having a positive and constructive experience, minimizing that which could cause a negative or unpleasant one. It is worth mentioning that, in certain therapeutic contexts, sometimes the objective is not to seek a "pleasant" experience, but rather a valuable or revealing one—even if this implies facing moments of difficulty (which do not necessarily imply something negative if they are well navigated and integrated afterward). In many cases, reports have associated these difficult experiences or bad trips with good long-term therapeutic results. This does not mean that anyone should look to have a bad trip, but it does mean that they can be a valuable part of the psychotherapeutic work and not necessarily be "bad" but rather "difficult" as explained previously.

Let's see the practical components in which all this translates.

MINIMIZING RISKS RELATED TO THE SET

The set is made up of the person and what they bring to the experience: their beliefs, expectations, mental and emotional state, concerns, intentions, state of physical and mental health, age, personality, and fears.

To minimize the risks in this area, it is advisable to:

- Learn about the substance and the experience very well, visiting risk reduction websites, reading books, watching videos, and so on. Some helpful materials are available in the Psychedelic Resources section of this book.
- Find out if you have any kind of family history of psychosis, bipolarity, or schizophrenia, and if you have ever suffered an episode or how you react to stress and lack of sleep. Psychosis and related conditions are very dangerous, and the use of psychedelics should be avoided at all costs if you suffer from any of them.
- Know your personality well and anticipate what your reactions might be in uncertain situations; if you have difficulty relaxing and letting go, if you tend to get anxious and need to be in control, if

you try to analyze and understand everything, if you have some degree of neuroticism—these are good characteristics to know about yourself beforehand.

- Learn tools and exercises to control anxiety, such as breathing, meditation, visualizations of quiet places, or yoga.
- Be aware of your own emotional state before starting a psychedelic trip, and try to start from a place of calm, well-being, and trust. It helps a lot to have a positive mindset[11] and choose a day when you feel especially well.
- Define a clear intention for the experience, but also know how to surrender and be open to whatever comes. Do not fight the experience, resist, or run away, as this often makes it more difficult or negative.
- Forget the routine concerns of the outside world—don't bring them along on the trip; you have to disconnect to be able to immerse yourself in the experience. It is important to have plenty of time for the experience and its subsequent integration without having to worry about the duration or upcoming commitments. At least have the day of and the day after the experience be free of commitments.
- Be ready to accept and surrender to the experience, whatever it may bring. You have to follow the classic psychedelic mantras: "trust, let go, and be open" to whatever comes, "turn off your mind, relax, and float downstream."
- Be patient with everything—with the preparation, the ascent, the psychedelic experience, and the subsequent integration. Rushing can greatly spoil the experience and turn it into an anxious one.
- If you feel like you are dying or going crazy, remember to keep calm and trust that this is part of the psychedelic experience and classic psychedelics (psilocybin, LSD, DMT) never killed anyone as far as we know, even at high doses (provided that no drug combinations or other extra risks are present).

---

11. Eline C. H. M. Haijen et al., "Predicting Responses to Psychedelics: A Prospective Study," *Frontiers in Pharmacology* 9 (November 2018): 897.

- Stay hydrated and nourished. During the experience, you may not feel thirsty or hungry, but the body still needs to drink and eat, so it is better to drink water and eat light meals, such as fruits, nuts, or juices, keeping in mind that food can decrease psychedelic intensity, especially with psilocybin.

MINIMIZING RISKS RELATED TO THE SETTING

The setting is made up of the physical, social, and cultural environment in which the psychedelic experience occurs. Like the set, it has a huge influence on its outcome and its risks. Therefore, it is just as important to pay close attention to the following:

- Choose a physical environment that is consistent with the intention of the experience. A recreational experience may be easier in a beautiful forest, while an introspective experience may be easier on a bed with eyes closed and headphones on.
- The physical environment must be safe, controllable, and predictable. It is better to avoid too many stimuli. Public places with a multitude of strangers, noise, and other variables that cannot be controlled are not a conducive setting for a good experience, especially first experiences. Instead, a house, a garden, or private spaces where things are under control are much safer, controllable, and predictable.
- The physical environment should be pleasant, comfortable, positive, and welcoming. Closely linked to safety, it is better to choose pleasant and positive spaces, which transmit good vibes, since uncomfortable or unwelcoming places can make negative sensations magnify enormously.
- Plan the session well in advance, leaving room for improvisation, but having everything you need close at hand (water, food, headphones, music, paper, notebook and pencils, paints) so you don't have to move around too much during the experience, since changes in space can totally alter the experience and not necessarily for the

better. It's also a good idea to chemically analyze the psychedelic substance beforehand at a risk reduction testing service.

- Music is a crucial element in guiding the experience with a positive and relaxing atmosphere. Changes in musical style can greatly affect the experience, so it is advisable to choose music that generates positivity and relaxation, such as the many playlists for psychedelic experiences available on Spotify and YouTube.

- Surround yourself with people you know well, trust, and whose good intentions you do not question, who are knowledgeable about psychedelics and do not make you feel judged. Any distrust, any suspicion or feeling of judgment can be magnified during a psychedelic experience and ruin it. In this sense, large groups are not usually a good idea, nor is consuming a psychedelic alone (especially the first few times). It's better to have a few trusted people (1–3) and preferably with experience and knowledge of psychedelics.

- When a few people are taking psychedelics at the same time, it's a good idea to have at least one person with psychedelic experience staying sober. That way they can look after the safety and wellbeing of the others and know how to help if someone has a difficult experience. The sober person who accompanies someone while they are in a psychedelic experience is known as a "tripsitter."

- It is also important that there is some freedom so that each person can choose their space based on their experience; that other people do not force anyone to be in a place where they do not want to be (unless for safety reasons), or to do something they do not want to do; that the intentions of those who take psychedelics in the same space be the same, compatible, or at least not get in the way. Ideally, you should be able to withdraw or remain silent if you don't feel like talking or interacting.

- If there is a guide or shaman, it is best to be attuned to their way of guiding or structuring the session. For example, if you are an atheist, a religious ceremony could be less engaging.

- Under no circumstances should you drive, operate machinery, handle dangerous objects, or carry out risky activities under the influence of a psychedelic.

But, if—despite carrying out all these risk reduction measures—a difficult situation arises, how should you act?

MANAGING "BAD TRIPS" AND
OTHER PSYCHEDELIC EMERGENCIES

Bad trips or difficult experiences are rare if the person has an adequate set and setting, but they could happen anyway, and it doesn't need to be too much of a concern if the person has only taken one psychedelic substance in not-so-high doses, is well accompanied and supervised, and if there are no other drugs, medical conditions, or other risks present. It should be remembered that the classic psychedelics (psilocybin, LSD, DMT) are pharmacologically very safe and there are no known deaths from their use, but the atypical psychedelics (MDMA, ketamine) can be dangerous at very high doses in certain people and contexts, or in combination with other substances.

People going through a difficult experience may feel very scared, anxious, confused, paranoid, afraid of death, or afraid of going permanently insane. Start by reframing the bad trip as a difficult experience that can be resolved; it is more accurate and better for the person going through the experience.

A difficult experience can be deeply unpleasant, but if someone is going through it, the most important thing to remember is that no one should panic, not the tripsitter and not the person going through the experience. As the saying goes, there is nothing to fear but fear itself. Keep in mind, these are only transitory experiences that do not usually pose a threat to the healthy individual, and with good management they can even be a good learning opportunity.

If the environment is not helping (noisy, messy, unfamiliar people, full of stimuli), it is a good idea to change it (quiet music, dim lights, fewer people, people who are trustworthy), or move the person to a better place, calmer and safer, with fewer stimuli. Avoid frightening the person by appearing nervous, scared, or worried, since it is very easy to involuntarily influence a person who is feeling the effects of psychedelics with our emotional state. It is advisable to convey confidence, that everything will be fine.

Remind the person who we are, where we are, and that they have taken a psychedelic drug voluntarily with a certain intention, and that what is happening is only a transient phase of the experience, that it is totally normal, and that although they may feel confused or scared now, they will soon feel fine or normal—everything will be back to normal soon. Remind them it is just a substance that their body is getting rid of, and the effects will not last long. In addition, these substances are almost not toxic, and no healthy individual has ever died yet just from consuming mushrooms, LSD, or other classic psychedelics alone. All the effects will eventually end.

Also remind them that they are not alone, nor will they be if they don't want to be, that you are by their side to take care of them and help them in everything they need. It is important that you do not touch the person without their consent, but if you do, it may help to hold their hand or rest your hand on their shoulder or a different part of their body that is not intimate or sexual.

It can be helpful to remind the person that their body is fine, that there is no threat, that things look fine from the outside and everything is temporarily in their head.

It is helpful to invite the person not to fight the experience, not to run away, but to surrender to it and flow with it, trusting themselves and the intention with which they took the psychedelic and trusting us as caregivers. Also invite them to focus on their body, on breathing, or on positive things, like thinking of a beautiful place, for example, to help redirect the experience toward a better phase.

Suggest that the person focus on their breath. Relaxation breathing techniques are often very helpful in reducing fear and anxiety.

If there is paranoia toward others, it may be beneficial to give the person some space in a comfortable, safe, and quiet area, but always supervised by the tripsitter, stating our intentions for them not to be scared.

If it is necessary to reduce the effects, a juice, smoothie, or little light food may help, as long as there is no risk of choking. For example, psilocin (the psychoactive compound from psilocybin) is removed from the body through glucuronidation, and this process could be supported by liver-healthy foods and nutrients such as sugars, curcumin, resveratrol, grape seed extract, milk thistle, hawthorn, omega-3 fatty acids, magnesium, apples, and kale. Consuming these foods could help to keep a healthy liver to speed up the body's ability to metabolize psilocin.

In the event the situation does not improve through these psychological interventions, or it worsens, and the person poses a risk to themself or others, emergency services can be of great help, providing medication in extreme cases, or if the situation is simply taking a long time to improve. The medications that are usually administered in this type of situation are anxiolytics, such as benzodiazepines (alprazolam or lorazepam), and in high-risk scenarios atypical antipsychotics (such as risperidone or olanzapine), but avoid haloperidol or other typical antipsychotics because they can aggravate the situation.

The decision to call an ambulance or transfer someone to a hospital should be weighed carefully in the case of difficult experiences that are not showing relevant physical or physiological risks for the individual or their environment. An unnecessary transfer could greatly accentuate the negative experience (noise, lights, unknown people, an ambulance, change of setting, a hospital, and questions).

If there is any risk to the life or physical integrity of the person due to previous medical conditions, inadequate dosage of the substance, combination with other compounds, error, or dangerous symptoms are manifested (tachycardia, hypertensive crisis, hyperthermia, coma or cardiorespiratory arrest), then emergency services should be immediately alerted, giving them the most precise information possible about the location, type of symptoms, substance that has been consumed, medication combinations, and other illnesses. In case of a purely psychologically difficult experience, however, it is better to work psychologically first with some of the ideas mentioned here to see if things improve before making the decision to call an ambulance or go to the hospital. It could be also helpful to ask the paramedics or ambulance team to avoid using the sirens or other extreme noises (if not essential) when approaching a person having a difficult experience.

In the hypothetical case that a person is unconscious, it is important to place them in recovery position and monitor their vital signs (breathing, pulse, blood pressure, temperature) while waiting for the ambulance to arrive. If the person is not breathing, cardiopulmonary resuscitation (CPR) maneuvers should be initiated. Fortunately, these types of situations are almost nonexistent in the informed use of psychedelics.

9

Conclusions:
Looking to the Future

In these pages, I hope I have managed to give you an introductory but comprehensive picture of this exciting process of psychedelic renaissance we are experiencing, and the enormous influence it could have in the field of mental health, society, and many other fields.

When I got interested in this field (almost two decades ago), and until just a few years ago, it was unthinkable to imagine such a hopeful moment in psychedelic research, or that it would have the health, sociocultural, spiritual, and even industrial repercussions it is beginning to have, or that it would open the therapeutic paths it is opening. It is indeed a cause for hope to the many people suffering from disorders that are so widespread in today's world, like depression, anxiety, post-traumatic stress disorder, and addictions. Moreover, at a time when our usual therapeutic tools are not being effective enough to tackle this epidemic of mental health disorders.

Despite the fact that, at first, it seemed that these substances were destined to revolutionize Western neuroscience and mental health therapies, ignorance about their use, together with their politicization, condemned them to the worst possible fate, their prohibition fifty years ago, taking away with it any potential clinical use. But, thanks to the courage and nonconformity of many people and to the new opportunities created since the end of the twentieth century, this field is now more alive than ever in the West (while it never disappeared in other places), not only in the field of basic research, but also clinical, with several substances already in very promising clinical trials.

At the same time (even before the restart of this research), many Westerners were already exploring on their own what the careful use of psychedelics could bring to various areas of their lives, testing them in a controlled way, in ceremonial, traditional, or private contexts, with the consequent increase in their popularity, rapidly changing the social perception of these substances, even becoming a trend in various communities. Currently, activist movements are managing to carry out popular local legislative initiatives to decriminalize psychedelics or even legalize access to them for medical purposes in several places of the world.

But it is also not convenient to get carried away by excessive optimism regarding psychedelics just yet. Although it is true that the results of its experimental use together with psychotherapy in controlled clinical contexts are very positive in many cases, we must remember that they are still, for the most part, studies with many limitations (carefully selected patients, with high expectations, in very controlled environments, difficult to blind[1]), and it is necessary to continue with increasingly solid research while slowly opening and expanding psychedelics' medical use, but with great caution before venturing into the implementation of widespread medical access. There is also not enough evidence yet to predict a great psychedelic future, as some would like to think, as these substances can be a powerful tool with a great impact on mental health, but they will not be a panacea. Additionally, we must not forget that its uncontrolled and uninformed use carries risks that should not be ignored as they once were, which led to the social misuse that ended in prohibition and the end of the first psychedelic renaissance.

Unfortunately, although psychedelic research is becoming more accessible every day and this is allowing its clinical development to accelerate, it is still not as easy as with other substances. This desire for progress often hits a wall of prejudice and bureaucratic obstacles

---

1. In a blind study, the patient does not know if they have been given the treatment or a placebo. It is very difficult to blind a study with psychedelics because their effects are so noticeable.

imposed by current drug policies, the same policies that prevented any developments in this field for decades, making it almost impossible to find financing due to scarce industrial interest.

For this reason, it is urgent to open an honest, unbiased, and well-informed debate on psychedelics and how to facilitate their research, development, and, most importantly, their safe and accessible implementation, which seems more than likely in the field of psychotherapy, but also in other potential fields. I was lucky to take part in this conversation at different forums, like the European Parliament, the European Medicines Agency, and even the United Nations, but many of these paths need a drug policy reform that eases the restrictions for research into the therapeutic applications of these substances and their mechanisms of action, as well as financing models that ensure not only quality research but also an agile development of the implementation of these therapies if, eventually, their effectiveness and safety are solidly demonstrated. Likewise, it is crucial to prevent the problems that may arise from their popularization outside the clinical setting through better dissemination of the knowledge of their risks and the development of risk reduction strategies by society, respecting the rights of traditional, cultural, and nonclinical uses while respecting individual freedoms, which should also be considered in this debate.

Regarding drug policy, it seems paradoxical that psychedelics, being one of the psychoactive substances with the least addictive potential, toxicity, and harm (in most cases without any reported deaths), and having enormous therapeutic potential, are de facto outlawed, being on the most restrictive international control list of substances; while other psychoactive drugs, without medicinal value, highly addictive, that cause a lot of damage, and that are behind the death of millions of people every year in the world, are fully legal and accessible to anyone of legal age, as is the case of tobacco (eight million deaths per year according to the WHO) or alcohol (three million deaths per year according to the WHO).

In fact, most of the time, the legal status of a drug does not correspond to scientific or objective criteria of its risk alone, but mostly to sociocultural and even moral criteria, and, in this sense, the case of psychedelics is especially striking if we compare its damage potential with its level of international control.

CLASSIFICATION OF DRUGS –
LEVELS OF HARM VS LEVELS OF CONTROL

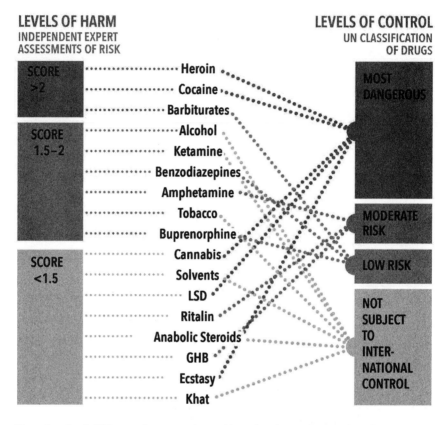

Harm levels of different drugs, evaluated by scientists, compared to their current international legal control levels. Psychedelics such as LSD or MDMA are in the lower part of the damage, but in the category of greater legal restriction. Image from David Nutt et al., "Development of a rational scale to assess the harm of drugs of potential misuse," *The Lancet* 369, no. 9566 (March 24, 2007): 1047–53; Nutt et al. and Gomis, Benoît, 2016, Modernizing Drug Law Enforcement, IDPC Drug Policy Guide-3rd edition (90–96) via The Global Commission on Drug Policy. (See also color plate 27.)

From the point of view of public health, drug policies should be based on scientific evidence and not on subjective or moral criteria. Truthful and objective information about drugs, as well as the basic principles of risk reduction, are crucial to be able to unblock this very harmful situation of social taboo that, based on misinformation, turns substances that could be very useful drugs for society into complete unknowns to the medical world, or even dangerous elements in the case of its uninformed recreational use.

In this sense, to avoid the problems that in the past accompanied the popularization of psychedelics, communication and scientific dissemination must continue to be rigorous, prudent, and well contextualized to avoid generating unrealistic expectations and a trivialization of the risks that can be associated with its poorly controlled use. This, together with a good knowledge of the substances, as well as risk reduction strategies, would largely mitigate the dangers that may be associated with their popularization, limiting the sensationalism or political instrumentalization that occurred in the past with these substances.

At the moment, we are not seeing many accidents or problems of great relevance associated with the use of psychedelics, largely thanks to the fact that, now, both researchers and society have a better understanding of the handling of these substances, but the great challenge for the future is to prevent the history of the last century from repeating itself.

In terms of financing this research, which is still so necessary, many of these psychedelic drugs are not of such direct interest to the traditional model of the private pharmaceutical industry since most are natural substances with low patentability margin or have an expired patent, while also being easy to grow at home and, in addition, they are only administered on a few occasions throughout a psychotherapeutic process, producing very long-lasting results. The business opportunity is not so much in the drug itself (as it happens in daily use treatments such as antidepressants and anxiolytics) but in the delivery method, the therapist, and the entire therapeutic process, which would force a reformulation of the traditional pharmaceutical and therapeutic model, including a shift in the biomedical paradigm in the approach to mental health.

However, outside the current model of psychedelic-assisted psychotherapy, there are other models where a more regular use of psychedelic substances could be implemented, such as their possible future use in promoting neuroplasticity or neurogenesis, in the prevention and treatment of neurodegenerative diseases through the use of microdoses, or new patentable psychedelic molecules, and that model of regular use could be more similar to a traditional pharmaceutical business model.

On the other hand, new biotech, pharmaceutical, and mental health companies are also emerging around psychedelics, successfully innovating and developing different models, thereby attracting more investment and research to the field, although not all of them are viewed favorably by the psychedelic community. However, public investment in the research and development of these therapies is more necessary than ever. After all, society and the national health system public coffers will be the main beneficiaries if this leads to advances in neuroscience and better treatments for mental health disorders in the population, especially if we take into account that these treatments could help many people with chronic disorders that do not respond to treatment, those who, in addition to the suffering that impacts them as individuals and their environment, also cope with work disabilities due to their mental health disorder, which entail a large expense for health services. All things considered, investment in psychedelic research could prove to be of tremendous benefit to public health, reducing the suffering of people with chronic disorders and saving health-care costs at the same time, because psychedelic-assisted therapies are intensive but much more cost-effective and efficient than conventional mental health treatments, and could also be an opportunity for preventing the development of mental health disorders in the first place.

But it is also crucial to consider the existence and expansion of the traditional uses in some cultures and the possibility that these practices could become restricted by the regulations for clinical use in Western medicine. These substances have been used for millennia, and it is precisely from this ancient experience that many of the principles used today in Westernized psychedelic-assisted psychotherapy have been derived. For our culture psychedelics may be something very new, but for many others, they are not new at all.

In turn, this last point opens up a debate that, little by little, is becoming more evident about whether the development of the medical use of these substances could also be extended in the future to "healthy" people (if we understand health only as the absence of disease) for preventive, spiritual, and self-knowledge purposes, in the face of existential crises, grieving, couple conflict, and other issues that could even sometimes develop into clinical conditions that need treatment. In short, nonmedical uses, which could also be of great social value and, although today they are far from being the priority of Western clinical research, have been part of the traditional and communal use of these substances for millennia, and would represent a paradigm shift in the approach to mental and community health in our societies that could even be understood as a preventive approach in mental health.

For all these reasons, just as it has been happening for some time with cannabis, disparities of opinion are also emerging within the psychedelic renaissance about what the eventual models of future access to these substances could look like and how to implement them, as well as its ethical, economic, commercial, and safety considerations. In this sense, it is very likely that more and more frictions will arise between players from different sectors such as research, industry, regulation, traditional uses, and even sociocultural contexts, because, although they all share the same interest in the potential of psychedelic substances, they don't always share the same ends or means—something that is already becoming clear in the context of the different models that have been outlined and supported by these players so far. There is a disparity of opinion regarding the development of popular legislative initiatives, patents on certain elements of psychedelics, the cultural elements of their use, the rights to access, who should be allowed to deliver these treatments, and even in the way of presenting news about scientific advances regarding psychedelics or their implementation on a big scale. Many of these possible models are already developing in parallel in different places, as is the case with the combination of the popular legislative initiatives for legalization in several U.S. states, combined with their current traditional uses for some communities, while the models of regulated medical access and pharmaceutical development keep advancing along a clinical development path.

In the medium term, the more than probable authorization of the medical use of MDMA for the treatment of post-traumatic stress disorder in many places (Australia already authorized it for special use in July 2023 and the U.S. will likely approve it in a couple of years when a final phase 3 trial is done) and of psilocybin for depression (which was also authorized for special use by Australia in July 2023 and may be approved in the U.S. in a couple of years) will join that of esketamine for depression (already authorized in 2019). These processes will be a real litmus test of the safety and potential of these substances, since it will probably be seen also as a great endorsement for their use outside clinical contexts. It will also test their level of acceptance in the medical community, in the psychotherapeutic field, in the press, and with legislators. At the same time, the psychedelic industry will continue with its projected growth and innovation regarding such a novel business that is arousing so much interest, with growth driven by frequent good news but also very exposed to bad news, as exemplified by the investment bubble burst of 2021 after the announcement of some not-so-amazing results in a clinical trial with psilocybin, or the impact of the first negative evaluation by the FDA for MDMA-assisted therapy for PTSD in 2024.

In short, the current psychedelic panorama is made up of many different actors and elements and, probably, there are still many more that will be revealed in time, so it is still early to predict the scope and future ramifications of this psychedelic renaissance, especially when more substances begin to be approved for medical use and their social popularity becomes mainstream. But, for the time being, it can be said that psychedelics are revolutionizing neuroscience. There is a lot of optimism and good prospects for their clinical use, and they garner more interest every day at an industrial, scientific, and sociocultural level. So, it does not seem risky to predict that, if the cards are played well and wisely, and research continues to show strong clinical potential, these substances could come to play an important role in the future of our societies.

We must be realistic and cautious in our optimism so as not to overestimate a phenomenon that, although it may become transcendental, at the moment it is only the brilliant promise of a better future for mental health and many other aspects of our society. However, we will closely follow the exciting advances that this psychedelic renaissance may bring us.

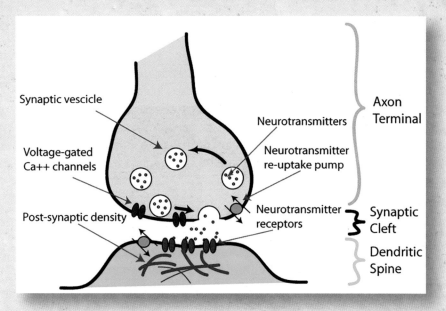

■ Plate 1. Simplified drawing of a synapse, where the axon of a neuron almost touches the dendrite of another neuron. Communication between the two is carried out by the release of chemical signals (neurotransmitters). Image by Nrets.

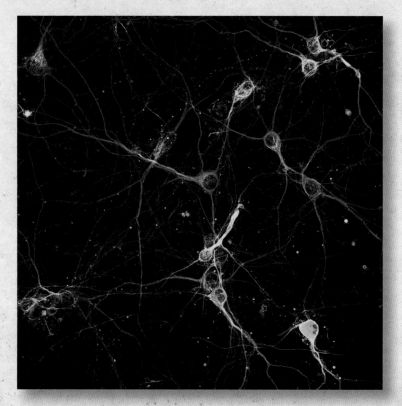

■ Plate 2. Network of neurons seen under the microscope. Image by ALoI88.

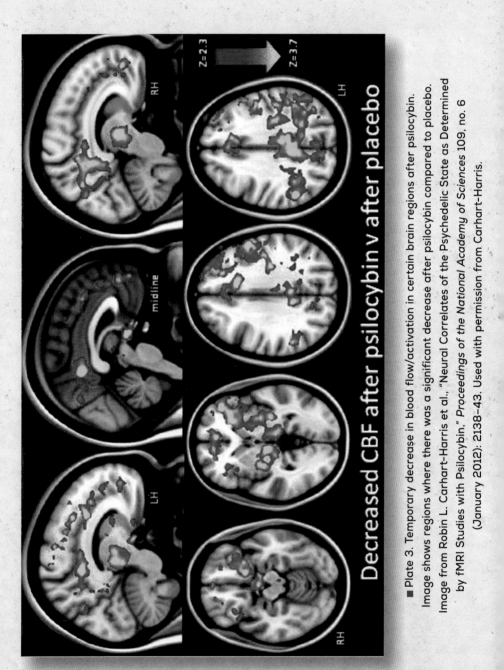

Decreased CBF after psilocybin v after placebo

■ Plate 3. Temporary decrease in blood flow/activation in certain brain regions after psilocybin. Image shows regions where there was a significant decrease after psilocybin compared to placebo. Image from Robin L. Carhart-Harris et al., "Neural Correlates of the Psychedelic State as Determined by fMRI Studies with Psilocybin," *Proceedings of the National Academy of Sciences* 109, no. 6 (January 2012): 2138–43. Used with permission from Carhart-Harris.

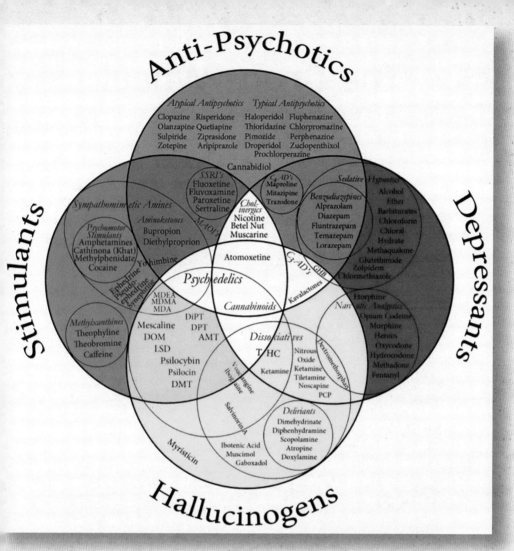

Plate 4. Venn diagram with psychoactive substances divided into four overlapping categories: stimulants, hallucinogens, depressants, and antipsychotics. Diagram by Derek Snider, 2005.

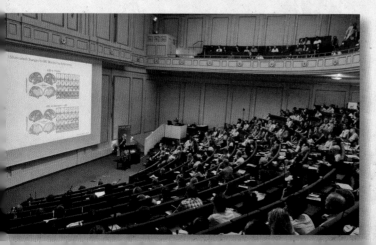

Plate 5. A growing number of annual scientific congresses are disseminating the latest advances in the use of psychedelics in psychotherapy, such as the INSIGHT 2021 Conference, in Berlin. Photo is the property of the author.

The Drugs Wheel
A new model for substance awareness

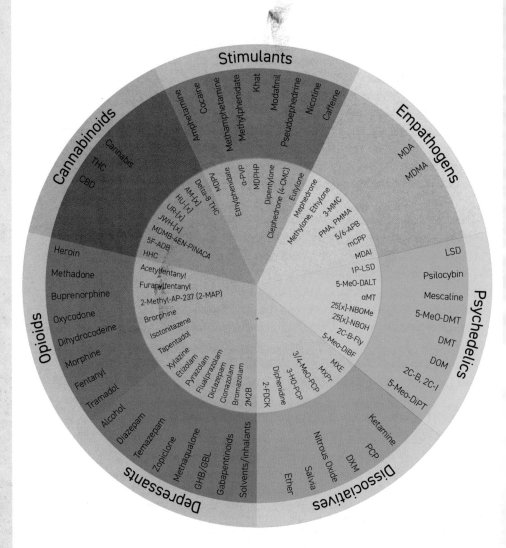

Outer ring: Established psychoactive substances

Inner ring: Newer psychoactive substances

In memory of harm reduction pioneer Dr Russell Newcombe (aka Dr Nuke)

■ Plate 6. The Drugs Wheel, showing seven drug classifications by their effects. Mark Adley, Guy Jones, and Fiona Measham, "Jump-starting the Conversation about Harm Reduction: Making Sense of Drug Effects," *Drugs: Education, Prevention and Policy* 30, no. 4 (2023): 347–60, via The Drugs Wheel website.

The Drugs Wheel

A new model for substance awareness

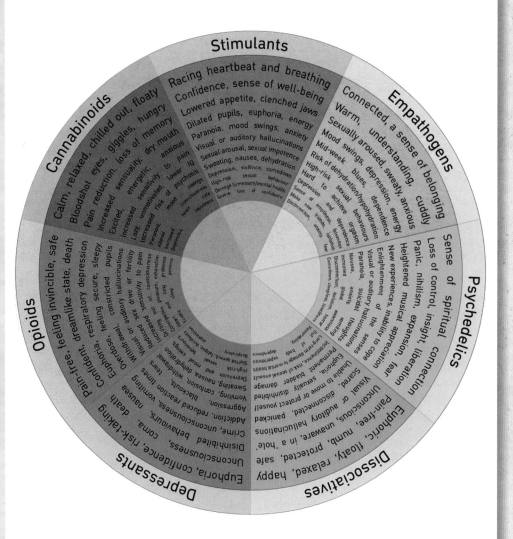

■ Plate 7. The Drugs Wheel, showing some detailed effects and some risks.
Mark Adley, Guy Jones, and Fiona Measham, "Jump-starting the Conversation
about Harm Reduction: Making Sense of Drug Effects," *Drugs: Education,
Prevention and Policy* 30, no. 4 (2023): 347–60.

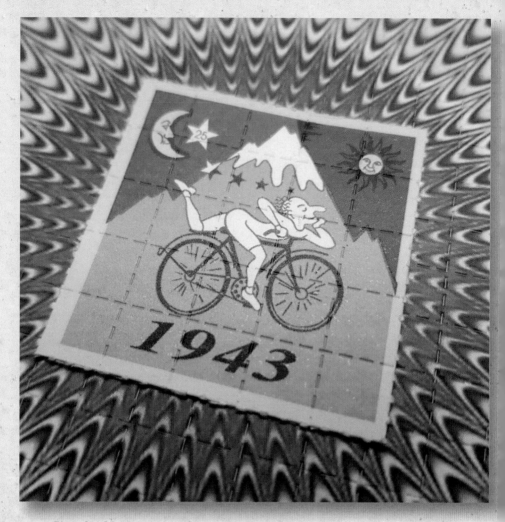

■ Plate 8. LSD blotter commemorating Bicycle Day: April 19, 1943. Each square of cardboard usually contains an impregnated dose of LSD that is usually between 100 and 150 micrograms, half of what Albert Hofmann took that day.
Photo sourced via the Blotter Store website.

■ Plate 9. Increase in Google searches for "psychedelics" between 2004 and 2024. Graph created by the author.

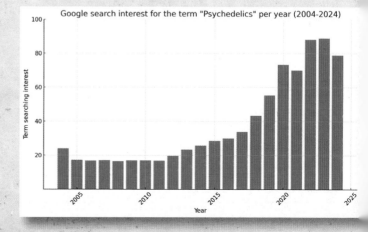

Google search interest for the term "Psychedelics" per year (2004-2024)

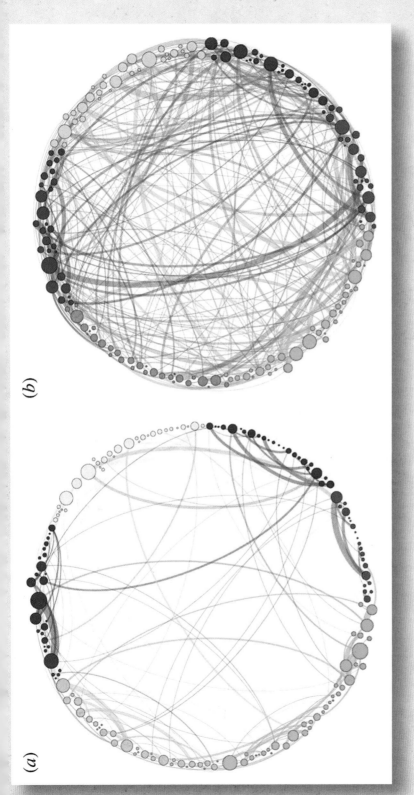

■ Plate 10. This representation shows the functional connectivity of different regions in a brain that has taken a placebo (a) versus a brain that has taken a dose of psilocybin (b). Image by G. Petri, P. Expert, F. Turkheimer, R. Carhart-Harris, D. Nutt, P. J. Hellyer, and F. Vaccarino.

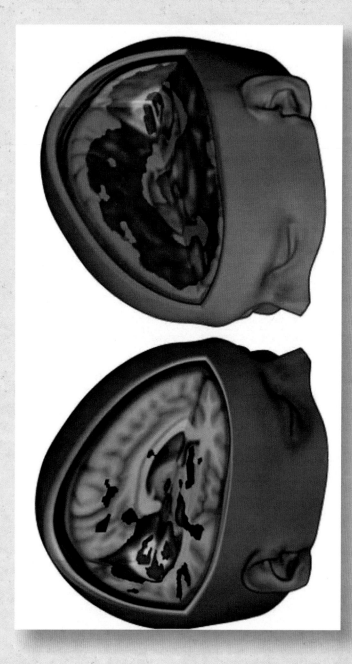

■ Plate 11. Imaging studies showed how LSD (right) increases connectivity between brain regions that do not communicate with each other under normal conditions (left). Image by Beckley/Imperial Research Program, from Carhart-Harris, et al., "Neural Correlates of the LSD Experience Revealed by Multimodal Neuroimaging," *Proceedings of the National Academy of Sciences* 113, no. 17 (April 2016): 4853–58. Used with permission from Carhart-Harris.

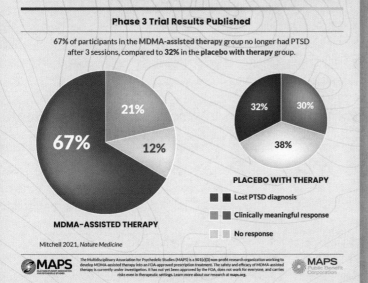

TREATING PTSD
WITH MDMA-ASSISTED THERAPY

Phase 3 Trial Results Published

67% of participants in the MDMA-assisted therapy group no longer had PTSD after 3 sessions, compared to **32%** in the **placebo with therapy** group.

67%
21%
12%

MDMA-ASSISTED THERAPY

32%
30%
38%

PLACEBO WITH THERAPY

- Lost PTSD diagnosis
- Clinically meaningful response
- No response

Mitchell 2021, *Nature Medicine*

MAPS — The Multidisciplinary Association for Psychedelic Studies (MAPS) is a 501(c)(3) non-profit research organization working to develop MDMA-assisted therapy into an FDA-approved prescription treatment. The safety and efficacy of MDMA-assisted therapy is currently under investigation. It has not yet been approved by the FDA, does not work for everyone, and carries risks even in therapeutic settings. Learn more about our research at maps.org.

MAPS Public Benefit Corporation

■ Plate 12. Graph representing the results of the study in the treatment group versus the control group. Sourced via MAPS.

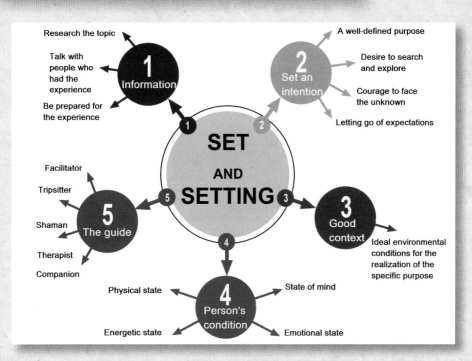

Research the topic

Talk with people who had the experience

Be prepared for the experience

1 Information

2 Set an intention

A well-defined purpose

Desire to search and explore

Courage to face the unknown

Letting go of expectations

SET AND SETTING

Facilitator

Tripsitter

Shaman

Therapist

Companion

5 The guide

3 Good context

Ideal environmental conditions for the realization of the specific purpose

Physical state

Energetic state

4 Person's condition

State of mind

Emotional state

■ Plate 13. Breakdown of the different variables of set and setting that should be carefully considered to reduce the risks when using a psychedelic.
Image by Jose Luis López Delgado via the Plantas Maestras website.

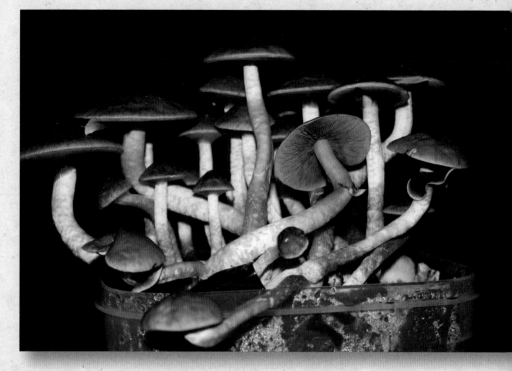

■ Plate 14. *Psilocybe cubensis* "golden teacher" mushrooms.
Photo by Mädi.

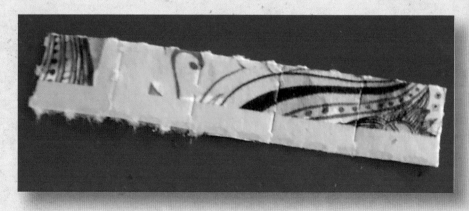

■ Plate 15. LSD blotter with five doses.
Photo by Motorbase.

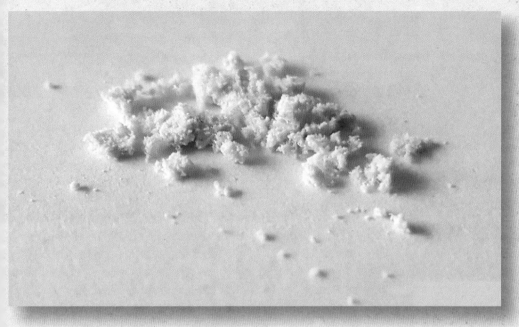

■ Plate 16. DMT in crystallized form, extracted from a vegetal source.
Photo by DM Trott.

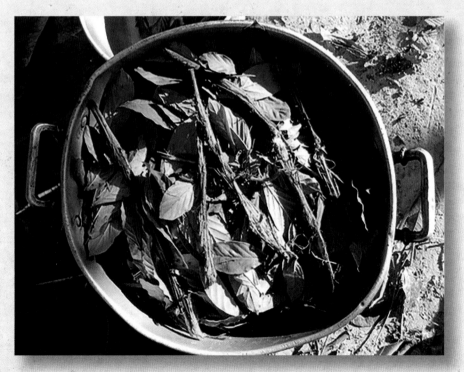

■ Plate 17. Ayahuasca ingredients before being cooked.
Photo by Awkipuma.

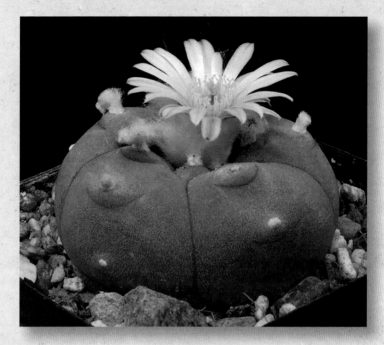

■ Plate 18. Peyote cactus in bloom, *Lophophora williamsii*.
Photo by Dav Hir.

■ Plate 19. San Pedro cactus,
Echinopsis pachanoi.
Photo by Forest and
Kim Starr.

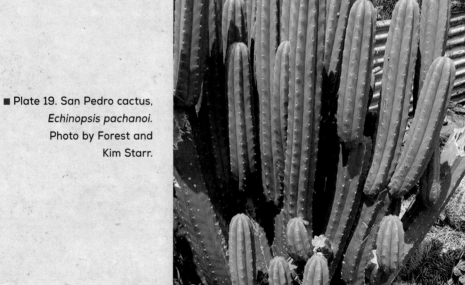

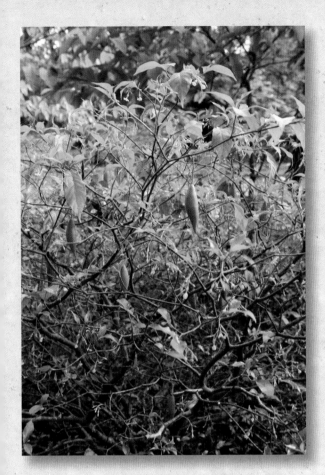

■ Plate 20. *Tabernanthe iboga* bush. Photo by Marco Schmidt[1].

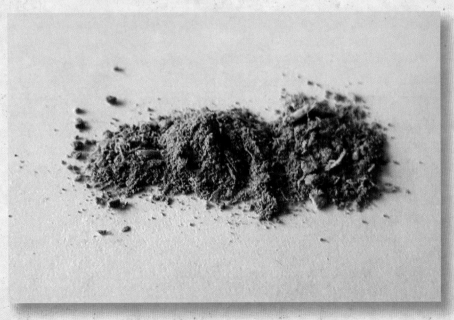

■ Plate 21. Iboga root bark powder.
Photo by DM Trott.

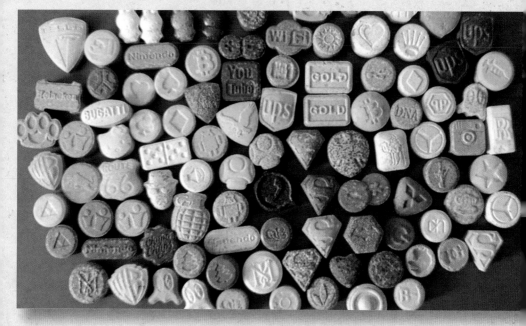

■ Plate 22. Ecstasy pills (MDMA).
Photo via the Rave Jungle website.

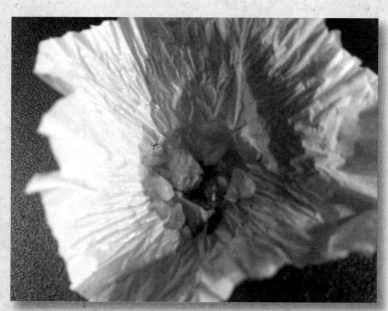

■ Plate 23. MDMA in
crystals.
Photo by unknown
author.

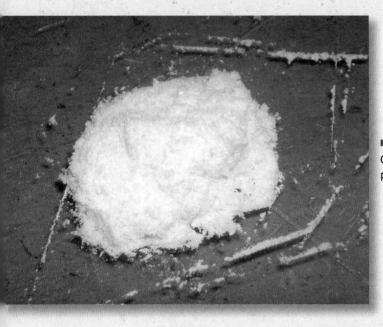

■ Plate 24.
Crystallized ketamine.
Photo by Coaster420.

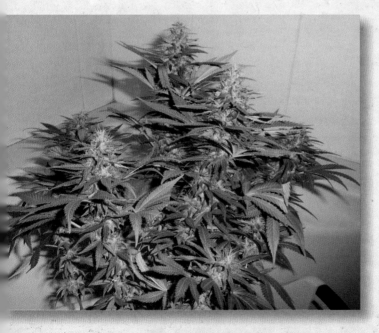

■ Plate 25. *Cannabis sativa* plant in bloom.
Photo by Pavel Sevela.

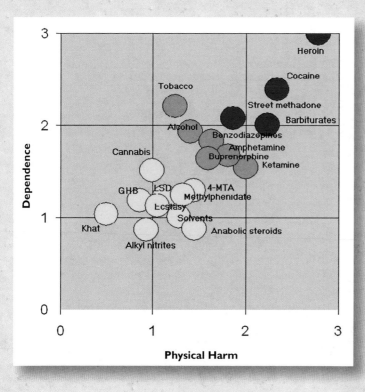

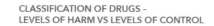

Physical Harm

■ Plate 26. Comparative table of the risks of different substances due to their physical damage and addictiveness; most psychedelics are in the lower part of both. A rational scale to assess the harm of drugs by Apartmento2. Data sourced from the March 24, 2007, article by David Nutt, Leslie A. King, William Saulsbury, and Colin Blakemore, "Development of a Rational Scale to Assess the Harm of Drugs of Potential Misuse," *The Lancet* 369, no. 9566 (March 24, 2007): 1047–53.

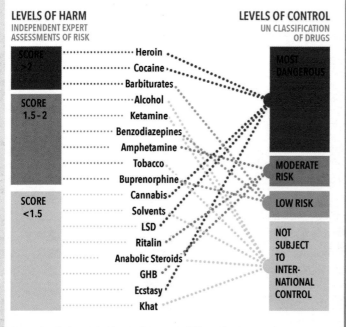

Sources: Nutt, D., King, L.A., Saulsbury, W., Blakemore, C. (2007); UNODC, Schedules of the Single Convention on Narcotic Drugs of 1961 as amended by the 1972 Protocol, as at 22 April 2017, and Schedules of the Convention on Psychotropic Substances of 1971, as at 18 October 2017

■ Plate 27. Harm levels of different drugs, evaluated by scientists, compared to their current international legal control levels. Psychedelics such as LSD or MDMA are in the lower part of the damage but in the category of greater legal restriction. Image from David Nutt et al., "Development of a rational scale to assess the harm of drugs of potential misuse," *The Lancet* 369, no. 9566 (March 24, 2007): 1047–53. Nutt et al. and Gomis, Benoît, 2016, Modernizing Drug Law Enforcement, IDPC Drug Policy Guide-3rd edition (90–96) via The Global Commission on Drug Policy.

Psychedelic Resources

INFORMATION ON PSYCHEDELICS
AND RISK REDUCTION

PsychonautWiki (psychonautwiki.org): Collaborative encyclopedia on psychoactive substances and psychonautics.

Erowid (erowid.org): Nonprofit harm reduction and educational resource with 60,000 pages of online information about psychoactive drugs and experiences with them.

TripSit (tripsit.me): Community focused on information on risk reduction and preparation of materials such as the Drug Combination Chart.

Drogopedia (ladrogopedia.com and @drogopedia): Website, YouTube, and social media channel providing drug and harm reduction education and information in short videos in Spanish.

RollSafe (rollsafe.org): Information and risk reduction resource focused on MDMA (Ecstasy).

TheDEA (thedea.org): Information and risk reduction resource focused on MDMA (Ecstasy).

Energy Control (energycontrol.org or energycontrol-international. org): Spanish organization dedicated to risk reduction and drug analysis at a national and international level.

Zendo Project (zendoproject.org): Part of MAPS, it's an organization that provides comprehensive and professional harm and risk reduction education and support to communities to help inform and transform difficult psychedelic experiences into opportunities for learning and growth.

Kosmicare (kosmicare.org): Portuguese organization dedicated to risk reduction, trip-sitting, and drug testing at music festivals and other events.

Drug Science (drugscience.org.uk): Independent scientific body in the United Kingdom. It works to provide clear and evidence-based information on drugs, without political or commercial interference.

The Drug Classroom (youtube.com/@TheDrugClassroom): Interesting resource with information on drugs.

International Center for Ethnobotanical Education, Research, and Service (ICEERS) (iceers.org): Research organization that has very good information on naturally occurring psychedelics.

PSYCHEDELIC RESEARCH

Multidisciplinary Association for Psychedelic Studies, MAPS (maps.org): A research and educational NGO, founded by Rick Doblin in 1986, that develops medical, legal, and cultural contexts for people to benefit from the careful use of psychedelics and marijuana.

Beckley Foundation (beckleyfoundation.org): Foundation focused on psychedelic research to drive evidence-based drug policy reform. Founded and led by Amanda Feilding in 1998 as a UK-based think tank and NGO.

International Center for Ethnobotanical Education, Research, and Service (ICEERS) (iceers.org): Nonprofit civil organization created in 2008 with headquarters in Barcelona and dedicated to promoting scientific research on plants with medicinal properties (including psychedelics) for use in therapies and personal development.

Heffter Research Institute (heffter.org): NGO that promotes research with hallucinogens and classic psychedelics, predominantly psilocybin, to contribute to a greater understanding of the mind and alleviate suffering.

Usona Institute (usonainstitute.org): An organization that supports and conducts preclinical and clinical research to improve the understanding of the therapeutic effects of psilocybin and other consciousness-expanding substances.

Center for Psychedelic & Consciousness Research at Johns Hopkins University (hopkinspsychedelic.org)

Center for Psychedelic Research at Imperial College London (imperial.ac.uk/psychedelic-research-centre)

Center for Psychedelic Therapies and Research (ciis.edu/research-centers/center-for-psychedelic-therapies-and-research)

INAWE Foundation (inawe.life): Non-profit organization that promotes innovation in mental health through the development of an ecosystem that facilitates the implementation of psychedelic-assisted therapies.

Sociedad Española de Medicina Psicodélica, SEMPsi (sempsi.org): Spanish Society of Psychedelic Medicine.

PSYCHEDELIC SOCIETIES AND OTHERS

Psychedelic Community (globalpsychedelic.org/locator): Directory of psychedelic societies around the world.

The Psychedelic Society (psychedelicsociety.org.uk): Located in the United Kingdom.

La Sociedad Psicodélica (lasociedadpsicodelica.es): Located in Spain.

La Sociedad Psicodélica de Madrid (facebook.com/PsychedelicSocietyMadrid): Madrid's Psychedelic Society.

PsychonautWiki Network (psychonautwiki.org/wiki/network): Directory with a large number of websites, organizations, and associations related to drugs in general and psychedelic drugs in particular.

RISK REDUCTION ORGANIZATIONS

Energy Control (Spain; energycontrol.org or international energy-control-international.org)

DanceSafe (United States; dancesafe.org)

Zendo Project (United States; zendoproject.org)

Fireside Project (United States; firesideproject.org)

Échele Cabeza (Colombia; echelecabeza.com)
Kosmicare (Portugal; kosmicare.org)
Check!n (Portugal; apdes.pt/en/portfolio/checkn-en)
Unity (The Netherlands; jellinek.nl/preventie/horeca/unity)
Techno+ (France; technoplus.org)
Checkit! (Austria; checkit.wien)
Safe'n Sound (Belgium; safensound.be)
Neutravel (Italy; neutravel.net)

DRUG CHECKING, TESTING, AND ANALYSIS

Energy Control Spain (energycontrol.org): Analyze drugs at their headquarters in Spain (Barcelona, Madrid, Antequera, or Mallorca) and at music festivals, nightclubs, or fairs.

Energy Control International (energycontrol-international.org): Analyze drugs for the whole world by mail.

DrugsData (drugsdata.org): Formerly ecstasydata.org.

WEDINOS (wedinos.org): A U.K. laboratory.

Pill Reports (pillreports.net)

Trans-European Drug Information network (TEDI) (tedinetwork.org)

ACTIVISM

Drug Policy Alliance (drugpolicy.org): Nonprofit organization based in New York City that seeks to promote policies that "reduce the harms of both drug use and prohibition and promote people's sovereignty over their minds and bodies."

Students for Sensitive Drug Policy (SSDP) (ssdp.org): International student activist organization that fights for drug policy reform and risk reduction policies.

International Drug Policy Consortium (IDPC) (idpc.net): Global network of more than 192 NGOs that promote objective and open debate on drug policies at the national, regional, and international levels. IDPC supports evidence-based policies that are effective in reducing drug-related harm.

Law Enforcement Action Partnership (LEAP) (lawenforcementac-tionpartnership.org): Formerly called Law Enforcement Against Prohibition, it is an organization that brings together police officers critical of current drug policy.

FORUMS

Reddit Psychedelics (reddit.com/r/Psychedelics): Reddit subforum focused on psychedelics.

Bluelight (bluelight.org): Dedicated to the discussion of risk and harm reduction strategies in everything that is considered a drug, such as a substance that alters the body or mind.

Drugs Forum (drugs-forum.com): Focused on discussion and support in addictions and risk and harm reduction.

DMT-Nexus.me (dmt-nexus.me): Forum and repository focused on DMT.

Cannabis Cafe (cannabiscafe.net): The largest Spanish-speaking forum for topics related to cannabis, psychedelics, and other drugs.

Shroomery (shroomery.org): Specializing in psychedelics, specifically in psychedelic mushrooms, also includes information about them.

Mycotopia (mycotopia.net): Specializes in psychedelics.

YOUTUBE CHANNELS

The Drug Classroom (youtube.com/user/TheDrugClassroom): Provides real education free of drug propaganda.

Psyched Substance (youtube.com/c/PsychedSubstanceChannel): Provides education on risk reduction and drug use.

Energy Control (youtube.com/c/EnergycontrolOrg): Channel with materials related to risk reduction, prevention, and information on drugs.

Drug Science (youtube.com/c/DrugScience)

Drogopedia (ladrogopedia.com): Website, YouTube, and social media channel providing drug and harm reduction education and information in short videos in Spanish.

PODCASTS

Psychedelic Times (psychedelictimes.com)
Psychedelics Today (psychedelicstoday.com)
The Third Wave (thethirdwave.co/podcast)
Psychedelic Salon (psychedelicsalon.com/podcasts)

SMARTPHONE APPS

TripSit Mobile: Risk reduction app from the TripSit association.
TripApp (tripapp.org)
KnowDrugs (knowdrugs.app)
Fireside Project (firesideproject.org)

NEWS AND CURRENT AFFAIRS

Sociedelic (sociedelic.com)
Psychedelic Spotlight (psychedelicspotlight.com)
Psychedelic Alpha (psychedelicalpha.com)
Double Blind Magazine (doubleblindmag.com)
Lucid News (lucid.news)
Psymposia (psymposia.com)
Revista Cáñamo [Hemp Magazine] (canamo.net)
Revista Ulises [Ulysses Magazine] (ulises.online)

DOCUMENTARIES ABOUT PSYCHEDELICS

How to Change Your Mind (2022)
Fantastic Fungi (2019)
Magic Medicine (2018)
The Way of the Psychonaut: Stanislav Grof's Journey of Consciousness
    (2020)
The Mind, Explained: Psychedelics (2019)
The Substance: Albert Hofmann's LSD (2011)
Psychedelia (2020)

María Sabina, Woman Spirit (1979)
Dosed (2019)
From Shock to Awe (2018)
Neurons to Nirvana: The Great Medicines (2013)
A New Understanding: Science of Psilocybin (2015)
DMT: The Spirit Molecule (2010)
Aya: Awakenings (2013)
The Sunshine Makers (2015)
Dirty Pictures (2010)
Journeys to the Edge of Consciousness (2019)
Hamilton's Pharmacopeia (multi-season documentary series)
The Last Shaman (2016)
Ayahuasca: Vine of the Soul (2010)
Entheogen: Awakening the Divine Within (2017)
Psychonautics: A Comic's Exploration of Psychedelics (2018)
Ibogaine: Rite of Passage (2004)
Peyote to LSD: A Psychedelic Odyssey (2008)
Science and Sacraments: Psychedelic Research and Mystical Experiences (2012)

MANUALS AND OTHER PUBLICATIONS

Manual of Psychedelic Support (psychsitter.com): The Psychedelic Support Manual is a comprehensive guide to establishing and managing support services for people who have difficult experiences with psychedelics at music festivals and similar events. The manual grew out of the work of the Kosmicare organization in Portugal, now joined by MAPS.

Psychedelic Library (psychedelic-library.org): Repository of all kinds of psychedelic publications.

Psychonaut docs (psychonautdocs.com): Repository of all kinds of publications for psychonauts.

Frequently asked questions about the psychedelic experience (erowid.org/psychoactives/faqs/psychedelic_experience_faq.shtml)

BOOKS

How to Change Your Mind: What the New Science of Psychedelics Teaches Us About Consciousness, Dying, Addiction, Depression, and Transcendence by Michael Pollan

The Psychedelic Explorer's Guide: Safe, Therapeutic and Sacred Journeys by James Fadiman

The Psychedelic Experience: A Manual Based on the Tibetan Book of the Dead by Timothy Leary

Psychedelics Encyclopedia by Peter Stafford

LSD. My Problem Child by Albert Hofmann

DMT: The Spirit Molecule: A Doctor's Revolutionary Research into the Biology of Near-Death and Mystical Experiences by Rick Strassman

Pharmacotheon by Jonathan Ott

Historia Elemental de las Drogas [Elemental History of Drugs] by Antonio Escohotado (in Spanish)

Historia General de las Drogas [General History of Drugs] by Antonio Escohotado (in Spanish)

Food of the Gods: The Search for the Original Tree of Knowledge— A Radical History of Plants, Drugs, and Human Evolution by Terence McKenna

LSD Psychotherapy: The Healing Potential of Psychedelic Medicine by Stanislav Grof

The Doors of Perception by Aldous Huxley

Acid Dreams: The Complete Social History of LSD—The CIA, the Sixties and Beyond by Martin A. Lee and Bruce Shlain

Your Psilocybin Mushroom Companion: An Informative, Easy-to-Use Guide to Understanding Magic Mushrooms—From Tips and Trips to Microdosing and Psychedelic Therapy by Michelle Janikian

The Psilocybin Mushroom Bible: The Definitive Guide to Growing and Using Magic Mushrooms by Dr. K Mandrake and Virginia Haze

Psilocybin Mushrooms of the World: An Identification Guide by Paul Stamets

PiHKAL: A Chemical Love Story by Alexander and Ann Shulgin
TiHKAL: The Continuation by Alexander and Ann Shulgin
Psychedelic Psychotherapy and Research. Past, Present and Future
  by Iker Puente

LEGAL INFORMATION

Release (release.org.uk/helpline)
ICEERS Ayahuasca Defense Fund (iceers.org/es/adf)
European Union Drugs Agency, EUDA (euda.europa.eu/publica-tions/topic-overviews/content/drug-law-penalties-at-a-glance_en): Comparative resource of approximate sentences for drug crimes in Europe, by country.
European Union Drugs Agency, EUDA (euda.europa.eu/publica-tions/topic-overviews/threshold-quantities-for-drug-offences/html_en): Comparative resource of approximate threshold quanti-ties that constitute different levels of drug offenses in Europe, by country.

OTHER RESOURCES

The wheel of drugs (thedrugswheel.com) by Mark Adley
The drug combinations chart (tripsit.me) by TripSit

The Legal Status of Psychedelic Drugs around the World

Francisco Azorín Ortega is a lawyer specializing in legislation and jurisprudence on drugs. The information in this appendix is as up-to-date as possible as of this writing. This information is subject to change.

I. INTRODUCTION

In order to talk about legislation and jurisprudence on psychedelic drugs, the first thing we have to do is define the latter concept. Although depending on how broadly the term is interpreted it may have different meanings, on this occasion we will use a fairly broad definition of the term. Such definition will include all those substances such as LSD, DMT, psilocybin, mescaline, and 2C-B that have perceptible effects on consciousness through, noticeably, acting on the serotonin 2A neuroreceptors, as well as other substances with more dissociative psychedelic effects, such as ketamine, which acts mainly on NMDA glutamate neuroreceptors. There are also other substances classified as empathogenic/ entactogenic, such as MDMA ("ecstasy"), with indirect interaction on serotonin 2A neuroreceptors, which many consider to be only semipsychedelic, but which in high doses can cause considerable psychedelic effects, like those caused by its sister substance, MDA[1], or 2C-B.

---

1. It was known in the popular slang of Spain in the 1980s and 1990s as "mescalinas" or "meskas" because of the similarity between its structure and some of its effects to those of mescaline, found in the San Pedro cactus and Mexican peyote.

It should also be noted that these psychedelic drugs can occur as isolated molecules (either extracted or synthesized), or as part of a plant or fungus (ayahuasca, psilocybe mushrooms, cacti, and the like), or even in some animals, such as the toad *Bufo alvarius* from the Sonoran Desert (Mexico), whose glands contain the most potent of the known psychedelics, 5-MeO-DMT. Although these toads were only recently discovered to contain this molecule, 5-MeO-DMT had already been synthesized in 1936 and isolated in 1959 from the seeds of the South American tree *Anadenanthera colubrina*. Another drug that is also found in animals is DMT. On top of being present in many plants, this molecule is also found in small amounts in humans and other mammals. It, therefore, seems that these compounds may be far more important to the workings of nature than we could ever have imagined.

Today, the Western world has far more psychedelics at its disposal than could have been available in the psychedelic boom era of the 1960s and 1970s, as well as in the "Second Summer of Love," which took place in Ibiza in 1987 and was exported to the United Kingdom between 1988 and 1989 with the emergence of the semipsychedelic MDMA and "rave culture."

The explosion of the phenomenon of new designer drugs, new psychoactive substances (NPS), and their sale on the internet, as well as the growing interest in shamanic cultures and their practice in Western territories, make it necessary to review and clarify the legislation and jurisprudence that tries to deal with this social reality. The presence of a certain sector of the population that uses these substances on an occasional or recurrent basis to navigate their consciousness, reconcile and accept their traumas, free themselves from their blockages, relieve their stress or depression, and, in short, try to live in this increasingly confrontational society more consciously and peacefully is becoming increasingly evident in our current culture.

The legal regime for psychedelic drugs around the world is a complex subject that has always been given to controversy and disparate interpretations, as well as constant legislative changes. In this appendix, I will attempt to provide as comprehensive and up-to-date a review as possible.

1.1 Why Were Certain Psychoactive Substances Banned?

The idea of banning all "recreational" use of certain psychoactive substances was driven by the growing influence of Anglo-American Christian Puritanism and the temperance movement against alcohol in the late 19th and early 20th centuries, which in the United States also led to the prohibition of alcohol between 1920 and 1933. The campaign for prohibition was also fuelled by racist sentiments towards immigrants from China and Mexico, who used opium and cannabis.[2]

In the 1960s, specifically in 1961, most countries in the world signed the Single Convention on Narcotic Drugs in New York, which banned opium, cannabis, and coca leaf, as well as their active ingredients and some derivatives (cocaine, morphine, and heroin). Later, new trends in the use of psychoactive drugs would emerge, such as the popularization of psychedelic substances, given that, in parallel to the promising clinical research with substances like LSD, psilocybin, and mescaline, some university professors such as Timothy Leary, writers such as Ken Kesey, and actors such as Cary Grant made their use fashionable in North America. This meant that the use of this category of substances quickly spread to the rest of the Western world, also playing an important role in the development of modern neuroscience.

With the upsurge of the nonclinical use of LSD, DMT, and psilocybin in the 1960s, associated with the hippie movement, the counterculture, and opposition to the Vietnam War, as well as their use in relation to some events reported in a very sensationalist way by the press, at the end of the decade, the United States decided to ban these substances. The first to do so was the state of California in 1966 when Ronald Reagan was governor, and they were later controlled at the federal level in 1969. Subsequently, in 1971, they were included in Schedule

---

2. Arbour et al. 2019. Classification of psychoactive substances. Geneva (Switzerland): Global Commission on Drug Policy. Report 2019. Retrieved from the Global Commission on Drug Policy website.

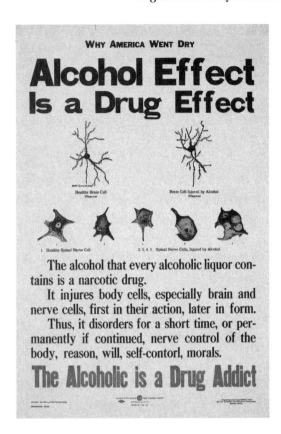

I of the International Convention on Psychotropic Substances, signed in Vienna, when Richard Nixon, the man who declared the so-called "war on drugs," was president of the United States.

In the 1980s, another of the world's most famous psychoactive substances, MDMA or ecstasy, came into vogue, being described as a semi-psychedelic and known for its entactogenic/empathogenic effects. It was banned in the United States in 1985 despite an administrative court recommendation to include it in Schedule III controlled substances, given that it is not very toxic and seemed to have psychotherapeutic effects. Despite pressure from some psychiatrists and other mental health professionals who used it for their treatments, the DEA (Drug Enforcement Administration) finally included it in its U.S. Schedule I classification, where the most dangerous substances with no recognized therapeutic value are placed, and in 1985 it was also included in Schedule I of the International Convention on Psychotropic Substances, which lists the most toxic and harmful substances considered to have little or no therapeutic value.

1.2 Criteria for Inclusion in One Control List or Another

Inclusion in one list or another does not always depend so much on the hazardousness or toxicity of the substance, or on its real therapeutic potential, but rather on a political or moral decision influenced by a given spatiotemporal context. In this regard, Nutt, King, and Phillips (2010) established a classification of the dangerousness of different drugs (legal and illegal) using a multitude of criteria, concluding that the least dangerous substances were psychedelic molecules, such as LSD and psilocybin, and semipsychedelics, such as cannabis and MDMA.[3] These substances were placed way below others, such as alcohol and tobacco, which, despite being more harmful, are legal.

In the words of an anonymous administrator and convention participant quoted by Mark Kleiman (professor of public policy and director of the Crime and Justice Program at New York University), ranking decisions are ultimately a consequence of the following premise: "If it's fun, it's Schedule One."[4]

1.3 The International Classification of Ketamine: A Substance with Recognized Medical Uses

The situation is different for ketamine, a substance with psychedelic and dissociative properties that was synthesized in 1962 by Calvin Stevens. Since then it has been used therapeutically in medicine and veterinary medicine as a general anesthetic and has also been included in the list of essential medicines of the World Health Organization (WHO) by virtue of its usefulness and safety. Since 2019, this substance, or rather one of its purified molecular forms (esketamine), patented by the pharmaceutical company Janssen

---

3. Nutt DJ, King LA, Phillips LD. 2010. Drug harms in the UK: a multicriteria decision analysis. The Lancet 376(9752):1558–1565.
4. Arbour et al. 2019. (See full reference in note 2 of this appendix.)

(owned by Johnson & Johnson), has been recognized by the FDA and other drug agencies for the treatment of depression, and, likely, this therapeutic indication will also be extended to racemic (classic) ketamine—though this has not happened yet.

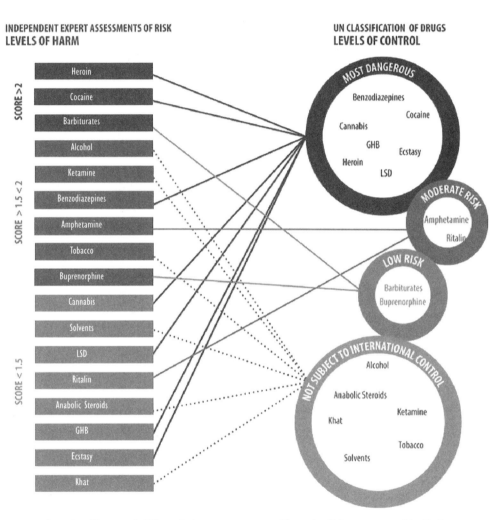

Levels of harm of different drugs as assessed by scientists, compared to their current international legal control levels. Figure adapted from: Nutt D, et al. 2007. Development of a rational scale to assess the harm of drugs of potential misuse. The Lancet 369 No. 9566:1047–53; Gomis B. 2016. Modernising Drug Law Enforcement. International Drug Policy Consortium, Drug Policy Guide, 3rd ed, 90–96.

Due to the rise of ketamine for recreational use, it was first controlled in the United States in 1999, and in 2006 it was listed by the United Nations Commission on Narcotic Drugs (CND) as a controlled substance under the 1971 Convention on Psychotropic Substances. Other states then transposed this prohibition into their national laws.

All the substances mentioned up to this point, except ketamine (which is in Schedule IV), are in Schedule I of the 1971 Convention on Psychotropic Substances where (according to the convention) the most dangerous and least valuable drugs in medicine are placed under control. Member states have also included them in the list where the most punishable substances under their respective national penal codes are to be found.

In the case of ketamine, this substance has always been recognized as having therapeutic properties as a general anesthetic and, more recently, as a psychiatric drug for the treatment of severe depression. For this reason, it has always been considered more therapeutic and less dangerous than other drugs; however, this cannot be considered scientifically correct since, for example, according to the report by Nutt et al. (2010), despite being below that of other legal drugs such as alcohol and tobacco, the harmful potential of ketamine for the individual and society is above that of LSD and psilocybin.

The WHO Expert Committee on Drug Dependence acknowledged that some concern had been expressed, stating:

> Placing ketamine under international control would have a negative impact on the availability and accessibility of this substance. This, in turn, would limit access to essential and emergency surgery, leading to a public health crisis in countries where no other affordable replacement anaesthetic is available.[5]

As can be seen, the case of synthetic drugs with psychedelic properties such as ketamine and MDMA or semisynthetic drugs such as LSD

---

5. WHO. 2012. WHO Expert Committee on Drug Dependence, Report No. 35, Technical Report Series 973. Geneva (Switzerland): World Health Organization, 9.

(derived from the ergot fungus) is not technically complicated when it comes to interpreting their legal status. As we will see below, legal interpretations become more complicated when dealing with plants or mushrooms that contain psychotropic controlled molecules.

The historical and legal arguments set out in the introduction to this appendix require us to navigate the paradoxical legislation and jurisprudence that regulate this issue.

2. STATES AND CITIES IN THE UNITED STATES THAT HAVE DECRIMINALIZED THE USE OF PSYCHEDELIC SUBSTANCES

2.1 U.S. Cities that Have Pioneered the Decriminalization of Psychedelic Substances

Since 2012, when the states of Colorado and Washington regulated access to cannabis for recreational use, there have been many efforts by associations advocating changes in current drug policies. To alleviate the great pandemic of mental illnesses that is increasingly present in society, such associations are seeking recognition of their therapeutic uses.

Thus, since then, not only has cannabis been regulated for recreational purposes in more than twenty states and Washington, DC, there have also been political and legislative movements to decriminalize the use of certain psychedelic substances in many parts of the United States, both at the state and municipal levels.

The first city to decriminalize the use of a substance other than cannabis was Denver, Colorado. In 2019, it did not quite legalize psilocybin (found in magic mushrooms), but it did, however, prohibit wasting police and judicial efforts to prosecute its use, thus being at the forefront of decriminalizing psychedelic drugs and recognizing their therapeutic value.

Other West Coast cities have also joined the reform, such as Oakland, California (historically very familiar with the use of entheogens), which in 2019 also decriminalized the use of plants, cacti, and mushrooms containing controlled substances such as psilocybin, mescaline, and DMT; and Santa Cruz, also in California, which in 2020 decriminalized the possession and cultivation of psilocybin-containing magic mushrooms, although the commercial sale of them remains illegal.

Washington, DC, followed suit in November 2020; and in 2021, the cities of Somerville, Bay State, and Cambridge, Massachusetts, did the same. Hence, we are no longer talking exclusively about cities on the West Coast. The decriminalization of psychedelics, like cannabis, has also reached the East Coast.

The latest cities to jump on the psychedelic bandwagon are Seattle and Port Townsend in Washington State; Arcata, Berkeley, Eureka, and San Francisco in California; Minneapolis in Minnesota; Evanston and Chicago in Illinois; Detroit, Ferndale, Hazel Park, and Ann Arbor in Michigan; Portland in Maine; Columbia in Maryland; and Amherst, Easthampton, Somerville, Northampton, Cambridge, and Salem in Massachusetts. These cities no longer prioritize the prosecution of crimes related to entheogenic plants. It, therefore, seems that, very soon, the possession and use of cannabis and other substances such as psilocybin (magic mushrooms) or mescaline (San Pedro cactus and peyote) will not be prosecuted in most states.

2.2 U.S. States that Have Decriminalized or Legalized the Use of Psychedelics

Regarding the decriminalization of psilocybin at the state level, the state of Oregon was the first to take the big step in November 2020, recognizing its use for therapeutic purposes, as it considers it useful for treating major depression and PTSD. Thus, possession of up to 12 g of magic mushrooms only entails a $100 fine or the completion of a health assessment. The possession of more than 12 g can lead to jail time. What is now completely legal in the state of Oregon is the provision of psilocybin treatments in specialized and certified centers. Colorado has decriminalized the personal use, possession, and private sharing of psilocybin and psilocin. This legislation also applies to the future inclusion of mescaline, ibogaine, and DMT, which will be considered for similar decriminalization after June 2026. However, retail sales of these substances are not allowed. The state plans to establish regulated "healing centers" where adults over the age of twenty-one can use these substances under professional supervision. These centers will offer a controlled environment for therapeutic use, but they are not set to begin operating until late 2024, with applications for licenses being accepted from that time.

The next state that seems to be getting ready to legalize the use of psilocybin for medicinal purposes is the state of California, where several proposals to legalize magic mushrooms' psychoactive molecule and other entheogenic plants for medicinal purposes have already been put forward. As of this writing, there are also such proposals in the states of New York, New Mexico, and New Jersey, and there are working groups studying legislative changes in at least ten other states.

2.3 Potential Problems Where U.S. Federal Law Comes into Play

Although these reforms are taking place at the local and state level, the United States is a federal republic, and U.S. federal law still includes psilocybin in its Schedule I controlled substances, which are considered the most dangerous and have the fewest therapeutic uses. This means that, even if they are in a city or state that has already decriminalized them, if a person is caught in possession of these substances by FBI agents, they can be charged with possession of illegal drugs under U.S. federal law.

2.4 Conclusion

In summary, since some American cities don't consider them to be harmful and do instead consider them to have increasingly recognized therapeutic value, they are no longer prioritizing the efforts of their local police to prosecute people who use this type of drug. However, the only state that has legalized psilocybin for medicinal purposes is Oregon, and the U.S. Congress, which legislates at the federal level on drug issues, is not yet in favor of legalizing such substances. Therefore, the reader of this book should take special care if in possession of a certain quantity of substances considered psychedelic, as, with a few local exceptions, they are still prohibited nationally and, of course, internationally in all countries.

3. GRADUATION OF PENALTIES FOR TRAFFICKING AND USE OF PSYCHEDELIC SUBSTANCES AROUND THE WORLD

In order to impose a penalty on the offender, drug trafficking offenses in countries that follow the rule of law are usually classified based on three basic factors: the alleged dangerousness of the substance, the quantity seized, and the aggravating circumstances of the case.

3.1 Increased Penalties for the Dangerousness of the Substance

In order to assess the criminal risks that would exist in cases of arrest for possession or sale of these substances, it should first be checked whether or not the member state in question is signed on to the 1971 United Nations Convention, whether or not it has also transposed the convention into national law (i.e., whether such signed international convention has been "translated" into national law), and finally, whether those particular substances are controlled in any of the schedules of the national drug law of each state.

> Despite this, there are countries with analogue laws: the US Analogue Substances Act, enacted in 1988, which automatically bans a substance if its structure and effects are "substantially similar" to those of an already banned drug; or the UK's Psychoactive Substances Act of 2016, which by default bans any psychoactive substance that by stimulating or depressing the person's central nervous system . . . affects the person's mental functioning or emotional state.[6]

Penalties are usually imposed according to whether substances are more or less dangerous to public health. Some countries such as the United Kingdom classify them in Schedules A, B, or C, with the

---

6. United Kingdom. 2016. Psychoactive Substances Act. London: Crown, paragraph 2. Retrieved from the U.K. government website.

most (officially) dangerous substances such as cocaine, heroin, LSD, and psilocybin placed in Schedule A, amphetamines and cannabis in Schedule B, and tranquilizers in Schedule C. The United States also has five schedules, included in the first schedule those substances that are allegedly most abused, most toxic, and not medically licensed (LSD, psilocybin, DMT, and 2CB), with ketamine, for example, being included in Schedule III, given it is medically licensed.

The case of Spain, for example, is more complex, having transposed the international drug conventions into domestic law by copying the same substances included in the schedules of the aforementioned international convention. Therefore, in the case of psychotropics, substances in Schedule I are officially more dangerous, and with less recognized therapeutic value, than those in Schedules II, III, and IV.

However, Article 36[7] of the Spanish Penal Code establishes a penal difference depending on whether or not the substance can cause serious damage to health. Paradoxically, however, this concept is not normative (not defined in the law), but jurisprudential (applied based on what previous judgments have interpreted), because the only drug currently classified by the jurisprudence of the Spanish courts as not causing serious harm to health is cannabis, and it is in Schedule I (the most controlled and with the least therapeutic potential) of the Spanish Narcotics Law 17/1967, while amphetamines and 2CB are in Schedule II (less controlled), although they are treated by case law as causing serious harm to health—yet another case of nonsensical legislation.

It should be noted that this jurisprudential concept, that of serious damage to health, is subject to change through the provision of pharmacological expert evidence, that is, what experts on the substance can say in court about its dangerousness. In fact, for example, MDMA (ecstasy) was considered by the Spanish National Court as a substance that does not cause serious damage to health in a hearing in 1994

7. Yoldi J. 1994 Jan 23. El éxtasis no causa grave daño a la salud según la Audiencia Nacional [Ecstasy does not cause serious health effects, according to the National Court of Spain]. El País (Madrid). Spanish.

in which the expert witness for the defense was Alexander Shulgin himself, considered the godfather or rediscoverer of this substance, as well as the mastermind behind the expansion of its use among the therapeutic community to treat post-traumatic stress disorder and other psychiatric illnesses. During the trial, the scientist compared MDMA to its chemical "big sister," MDA, to explain that MDMA is less neurotoxic than MDA and that it does not have high addictive power. Thanks to testimony, the court decided to consider ecstasy a substance that does not cause serious damage to health (Yoldi 1994) and was therefore made punishable by a lesser penalty than cocaine and LSD. However, later on, Spanish court jurisprudence changed its opinion, considering ecstasy (MDMA) a health hazard. This was possibly due to the Leah Betts scandal, the eighteen-year-old British girl who died after taking an ecstasy pill at a house party with her parents. During the days when she was in a coma, a media campaign made the front page of newspapers in the United Kingdom and around the world, publishing photos of her on her deathbed and filling the streets up with pictures of her face accompanied by messages about the dangers of drugs. Later, the doctor who treated her said that she had died from overhydration, known as hyponatremia, as she drank too much water in an attempt to quash the effect of the pill. In reality, deaths from ecstasy use are not common and occur much less frequently than those related to alcohol or tobacco,[8] without resulting in the criminalization of their possession or distribution.

3.2 Increasing Penalties for Quantity Seized

The different countries that have banned the possession and sale of different psychedelic (or other) drugs also tend to establish tables to increase penalties according to the quantity of the substance seized.

This is the case, for example, in the United States, which has tables of equivalence between substances in which, if a certain quantity is exceeded,

---

8. Collin M. 2002. Estado alterado: la historia de la cultura del éxtasis y del acid house [Altered state: the history of ecstasy culture and "acid house"]. Barcelona (Spain): Alba Editorial. Spanish.

the minimum or maximum penalty required by federal law is increased. In the case of ecstasy, for example, there is a table of equivalence concerning cannabis, with the equivalence being 1–500. This means that 1 g of MDMA is equivalent to the penalty for 500 g of cannabis. This equivalence was raised in 2001 from 35–1 to 500–1, but in 2011, with the collaboration of the Multidisciplinary Association for Psychedelic Studies (MAPS), it was set by two American courts at 200–1, considering that the scientific reports provided in 2001 were based on exaggerated, and scientifically unsound, perceptions of the harmfulness of MDMA, and that MDMA was no more harmful than cocaine. In 2017, an attempt was made to reclassify the equivalence of ecstasy in a proceeding in which Dr. Rick Doblin, the founder of MAPS, was an expert witness, without succeeding in having the dangerousness of MDMA reconsidered.[9] However, with the work of people like Doblin and MAPS, MDMA is now in phase 3 clinical trials, and FDA recognition for the treatment of post-traumatic stress disorder and other psychiatric illnesses is expected by 2024.

3.3 Increased Penalties for Aggravating Circumstances

Penalties are also often increased for other aggravating circumstances, such as committing a crime with violence, belonging to a criminal organization, or trafficking minors.

Sentences for drug trafficking are typically set at between two and ten years in most countries, rising to twenty years or even life imprisonment in countries such as the United States or the United Kingdom, when there are very special and specific circumstances such as the use of criminal gangs or violence. There are regions where sentences can be particularly high, such as Africa, the Middle East, and Asia.

3.4 Tolerance in Cases of Small Quantities for Personal Use

In most European countries, some U.S. states, Canada, and in most South American countries, drug use for personal use is tolerated, and offenses

---

9. Multidisciplinary Association for Psychedelic Studies USSC Testimony re: MDMA March 15, 2017.

for simple possession of drugs are usually punishable by a prison sentence of between six months and two years, which may be suspended if the offender is a first offender (no previous criminal record) or undergoing drug detoxification treatment. It might also just be replaced by a fine.[10]

However, the specific legislation in each country needs to be studied in detail to find out whether there is a law for minimum dose for personal use or whether simple possession is punishable by administrative fines and the like.

3.4.1 Latin American Countries

Latin American countries such as Colombia, Uruguay, Peru, and Mexico have minimum personal dose laws, in which small quantities of various substances cannot even be punished by an administrative rule.

In Peru, for example, drug trafficking is punishable by a sentence of eight to fifteen years, and possession for the purpose of trafficking is punishable by six to twelve years, and even life imprisonment if forced by violence or intimidation to plant drugs. However, possession for the personal use of up to 5 g of cocaine base paste, 2 g of cocaine hydrochloride, 8 g of marijuana, and 2 g of its derivatives, or 250 milligrams of MDMA or similar substances[11] is not criminalized. Having said this, it seems that the dose is seized even if it is not sanctioned in all countries except Uruguay.[12]

In Mexico and Colombia, for example, the constitutional courts have issued two rulings, on November 4, 2015, and June 6, 2019, respectively, in which, in the section on the weighing of affected fundamental rights

---

10. Cavada JP. 2020. Criterios para el sancionamiento del consumo o tráfico de drogas en el derecho extranjero [Criteria for the punishment of drug use or trafficking abroad]. Santiago de Chile: Biblioteca Nacional del Congreso de Chile. Spanish. Retrieved from the Biblioteca Nacional del Congreso de Chile website.

11. Martín A, Muñoz J. 2019. El estatuto legal de la ayahuasca en España: la relevancia penal de los comportamientos relacionados con su consumo y posesión [Legal status of ayahuasca in Spain: the criminal relevance of behaviors related to its consumption and possession]. Valencia (Spain): Tirant lo Blanch. Spanish.

12. Salvo Uruguay, dosis mínima se incauta en toda A. Latina [With the exception of Uruguay, minimum doses are seized throughout Latin America]. El Nuevo Siglo (Bogotá, Colombia) 2018 Sept 6. Spanish.

and collective legal interests to be protected (public health and safety), it is concluded that these two collective interests should not prevail over the individual freedom and free development of the personality of the drug user, as long as the test of proportionality in the interpretation of these affected fundamental rights and protected legal interests is not passed. In other words, individual liberties prevail over the personal consumption of substances in the face of other considerations, such as public health and safety, allegedly threatened by personal drug consumption. However, the Colombian Constitutional Court had already declared the criminalization of drug use unconstitutional in Ruling C-221/94. Despite this ruling almost two decades ago, subsequent governments have criticized this judicial decision and attempted to recriminalize drug use for personal consumption, generating laws that currently prohibit use but do not criminalize it. This ruling was used by academic researchers and by countries such as Switzerland and the Netherlands to adapt their arguments for their legislation.[13]

In Argentina, penalties range from one month to two years imprisonment, plus a fine for possession for personal use (Art. 14, second paragraph, Law 23.737); from one to six years imprisonment, plus a fine for simple possession (first paragraph of the same article); and from four to fifteen years imprisonment, plus a fine for possession for commercial purposes (5 inc. C of the same law). The latter Article 5 also establishes penalties for trafficking of four to fifteen years imprisonment, plus a fine, and some aggravating circumstances are described in subsequent articles. Cross-border trafficking is punishable under the Customs Code (Art. 866), with penalties ranging from four and a half months to sixteen years.

3.4.2 The Spanish Case

In Spain, as long as no specific quantities of psychedelics are found that exceed what is considered usual for daily personal use for three to five days, and provided there are no indications of trafficking (such as having

---

13. Uprimny R. 2019. A 25 años de la sentencia C-221/94 en Colombia: una oportunidad perdida [Twenty-five years after the C-221/94 sentence in Colombia: a missed opportunity]. London: International Drug Policy Consortium. Spanish. Retrieved from the International Drug Policy Consortium website.

the substance divided into doses, having a precision scale, a multitude of substances, a notebook with notes, cash, and so on), the case would not be sent to a criminal court. This has been established by the National Institute of Toxicology at a maximum of 2.4 g of pure MDMA or 0.003 g of LSD,[14] with a fine of between 601 and 30,000 euros[15] being imposed in these cases. However, this law is to be amended shortly, and it seems that fines for simple possession will be considered minor (the amount would be between 100 and 600 euros), and consumption on public roads will be punished with a fine of 601 euros.[16] However, perhaps because they are less prevalent in the population, substances such as psilocybin are not included in this table of quantities regarding personal consumption, nor do they appear in tables in other countries. In this case, and in order to calculate the dose that could be regarded as for personal use, and what quantities could be considered as trafficking and therefore subject to higher penalties, ad hoc expert evidence will be required. Despite exceeding the National Institute of Toxicology (INT) quantities, Spanish jurisprudence requires proof of intent to traffic the substance to convict through other evidence or indications.

To further highlight the lack of solid scientific criteria when establishing penalties for drug trafficking in Spain, we can recover this excerpt from an article on the words spoken by the director of INT at the time of issuing the famous report:

> "That table was part of a technical report that was sent in 2001 to the Supreme Court, but at no point did we address whether they should be used to set sentences or not," Gómez explained. Gómez agreed with the opinions of other experts consulted, and clarified that "the effect of a toxic substance on the organism depends

---

14. Instituto Nacional de Toxicología (2001). Informe sobre dosis mínima psicoactiva, de 18 de octubre de 2001 [Report on minimum psychoactive dose, October 18, 2001]. Madrid: Instituto Nacional de Toxicología. Spanish.

15. Ley Orgánica 4/2015, de 30 de marzo, de protección de la seguridad ciudadana [Organic Law 4/2015, March 30, on the protection of public safety]. Published in BOE [Official State Bulletin] No. 77, March 31, 2015. Spanish.

16. Azorín F. 2021 Dec 14. Reforma de la Ley Mordaza y cannabis: es urgente [Reform of the "Gag Rule" and cannabis: it's urgent]. El Salto (Madrid). Spanish.

on the person, their size, their state and how used to it they are. It is the same as with Valium which doesn't have the same effect on everyone. Some people fall asleep with one pill, others don't feel anything when they take two."[17]

In other words, not even the authors of the report considered it fair that sentences should be passed based on this technical report. As historically only a summary table has been available on the internet, I requested the report via Spain's Transparency Portal. It came as a great surprise to see that there were no bibliographical references that could be refuted by other experts through contradictory expert evidence. Only a legend full of scientific and logical deficiencies could be found. For example, all substances have a range of daily doses, and to obtain the maximum amount for personal use, the highest end of the range is multiplied by 5 (in reference to five days of personal use). However, in the case of MDMA (ecstasy), it is stated that between one and fifteen tablets of 80 mg can be consumed per day when, according to the report, the norm is to take six tablets per day (which goes against the logic of the table, which always multiplies by 5 the highest dose of the range).

3.4.3 Personal Use Doses for Non-Scheduled Substances
In those cases where the substance in question does not appear in the table, it is up to the police to decide whether, depending on the dose seized, a case should be dealt with under criminal or administrative law. However, as we have said, the tables are not complete and do not cover the full range of psychopharmacological drugs used by people who consume illegal substances. In fact, in the case of psilocybin mushrooms, there is an acquittal in Spain that states the following:

In the specific case of the ruling, 670 mushrooms weighing 202.5 grams were seized. In this sense, the minimum active dose

---

17. Lázaro JM, De Benito E. 2004 Apr 11. Toxicología se desmarca del baremo que utiliza el Supremo para condenar a 'camellos' [Toxicology disassociates itself from the scale used by the Supreme Court to sentence "dealers"]. El País (Madrid). Spanish.

[of pure psilocybin] is around 2 milligrams, 10 to 20 milligrams is a medium dose, and a high dose is 30 milligrams or more. The effects of medium doses last for 4 to 6 hours and those of high doses for up to 8 hours. Based on these parameters, the daily dose of [pure psilocybin] consumption can be put at around 100 mg. If we multiply this amount by 1.7 mg of psilocybin per mushroom, the result is just over 1 gram of this substance [pure psilocybin]. This is an amount that guarantees consumption for about 10 days.[18]

The reader will note, if experienced in the use of mushrooms, that, when it comes to psychedelics such as mushrooms or LSD, which are usually taken very infrequently, in annual or monthly doses at most, this ruling does not make much sense. However, drug jurisprudence is often constructed by people with little knowledge of the subject who assume that everyone who takes drugs is addicted and that taking a substance necessarily implies continuous use throughout the day to be under its effects twenty-four hours a day, every day. This flawed logic is probably derived from the problematic use of certain highly addictive opiates, such as heroin.

3.4.4 The Dutch Case

In the Netherlands, for example, possession of up to 5 g of fresh mushrooms and 0.5 g of dried mushrooms used to be tolerated, but in 2008, fresh mushrooms were explicitly banned. Previously, only dried mushrooms were considered to be "a preparation containing psilocybin" as defined by the 1971 Psychotropic Convention. Since 2008, the market switched from mushrooms to psilocybin-containing truffles, given that these fungal species were not explicitly controlled.[19]

3.4.5 Portugal and Its Risk and Harm Reduction Policy

Another country where possession of drugs for personal use is not criminalized is Portugal. Law 30/2000, adopted in November 2000

---

18. Sentence from the Audiencia Provincial of Alicante No. 129/2013 February 28.
19. Legal situation of psilocybin mushrooms. Obtained from Wikipedia.

and enforced since July 2001, decriminalized the consumption, acquisition, and possession of drugs for personal use. A decree establishes the quantities that will not lead to criminal prosecution for each substance, estimating as a maximum the daily consumption of a drug for a period of ten days. If someone is caught consuming in the street, they are given the option of attending an interview with a committee comprised of a psychologist, a social worker, and a jurist so that they can analyze whether the situation is considered problematic consumption and, if so, offer the consumer therapeutic help (Cavada 2020).

3.4.6 France and Italy and Their Hardline Drug Policy
France, for its part, has always been a very belligerent country on drug issues within Europe. However, penalties for simple possession are less than one year, plus a fine, and the offender is usually required to attend and pay for a drug awareness course (Cavada 2020).

Italy is another country that establishes higher penalties for drug trafficking offenses, especially if committed by organized mafias. In terms of penalties for simple possession, it is also a rather tough country because, even if criminal proceedings are not initiated, serious administrative sanctions, such as the loss of one's driver's license, could be imposed. The country also offers substitution treatments for confiscations where no evidence of drug trafficking exists.[20]

3.4.7 Other European Countries
Concerning the tables of doses for personal use in other European countries, the European Union Drugs Agency (EUDA) produces summary tables for each country, available in the "Publications" section of the EUDA website ("Threshold quantities for drug offences").

3.5 Conclusion
In conclusion, in most countries that have a legal system based on the rule of law, with constitutions that protect and recognize fundamental rights of the individual, simple possession of drugs for personal use is

---

20. Cavada JP. 2020. (See full reference in note 10 of this appendix.)

not usually punishable by imprisonment. And if a prison term for personal use is stated in the law, it is usually symbolic and probably will be suspended if the person is a first offender or undergoes drug treatment. However, each factual situation can be interpreted in different ways, depending on the case, so to minimize the legal risks of possession and use, the drug user should do his or her part to understand how the supposed tolerance of personal possession for the personal use of drugs is interpreted in the legal practice of the relevant country.

3.6 Special Caution in Countries with Strict Drug Laws

In some countries around the world, especially in Africa, the Middle East, and Asia, what we in the West would call a "rule of law with due process and recognition of individual rights" is not strictly enforced. Therefore, drug possession in countries such as the Philippines, China, India, Malaysia, Qatar, Saudi Arabia, and others can lead to very serious problems with the law. Paradoxically, it seems that Thailand,[21] one of these countries, intends to regulate recreational cannabis soon, having regulated access to the plant for medicinal purposes in 2020. It seems that drug policy is changing dramatically in some countries, and not necessarily only in Western ones or those with a democratic culture that, through the rule of law, recognizes the individual's fundamental rights.

4. INTERNATIONAL CONTROL OF PLANTS CONTAINING MOLECULES CLASSIFIED AS PSYCHOTROPIC UNDER THE 1971 CONVENTION

As mentioned above, when we encounter interceptions of plant or fungal substances containing a molecule classified as psychotropic under the 1971 Convention on Psychotropic Substances, the legal interpretation becomes quite complicated.

---

21. Tailandia, primer país de Asia que despenaliza la marihuana [Thailand, the first country to decriminalize marijuana]. Diario Las Américas (Miami, FL) 2022 Jan 25. Spanish.

4.1 The International Narcotics Control Board's Interpretation of the Conventions

In this section, we will analyze the thesis of the International Narcotics Control Board (INCB) when applying the international conventions to certain psychoactive plants that are not expressly controlled but contain substances that are.

The INCB or NCBI, in its 2010 and 2012 reports, states that there are only three plants controlled by the international drug conventions. These are only the cannabis plant (*C. sativa*); the coca leaf (*Erythroxylum coca*), from which cocaine is extracted; and the white poppy (*Papaver somniferum*), from which the opium needed to make morphine and heroin is extracted. In other words, the 1961 Convention on Narcotic Drugs only banned certain plants.

Although some active ingredients with stimulant or hallucinogenic effects contained in certain plants are controlled under the 1971 Convention, no plants are currently controlled under that convention or the 1988 Convention. Nor are preparations (e.g., decoctions for oral consumption) made from plants containing such active ingredients under international control.

Examples of such plants or plant materials are khat (*Catha edulis*), whose active ingredients cathinone and cathine are included in Schedules I and III of the 1971 Convention; ayahuasca, originating in the Amazon basin, mainly consisting of a preparation of *Banisteriopsis caapi* (a jungle vine) and another tryptamine-rich plant (*P. viridis*) that contains various psychoactive alkaloids such as DMT.[22]

No plants, even those containing psychoactive ingredients, are currently controlled under the 1971 Convention, although in some cases the active ingredients they contain may be under international control. For example, cathine and DMT are psychotropic substances listed in Schedule I of the 1971 Convention, while the plants and herbal preparations containing them, namely khat and ayahuasca, respectively, are not subject to any restriction or control measures.[23]

---

22. International Narcotics Control Board. 2011. 2010 Report. United Nations. New York.
23. International Narcotics Control Board. 2013. 2012 Report. United Nations. New York.

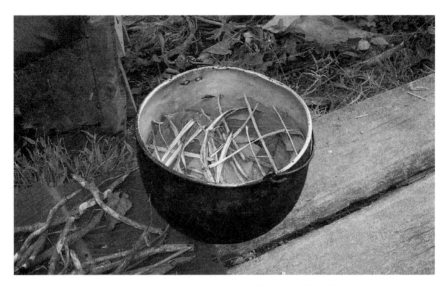

Ayahuasca, ready to be cooked. Photo by Terpsichore.

4.2 Possibility of Some Countries Controlling Certain Psychoactive Plants on an Individual Basis

Despite the explanation in the previous section, there may be countries that have expressly prohibited plants or parts of plants, as is the case in France and Italy with ayahuasca and in the Netherlands with magic mushrooms.

However, despite the interpretations of the International Narcotics Control Board, the truth is that, in most countries, seizures of ayahuasca are indeed reported and the police do usually confiscate magic mushrooms.

In Spain, most of the judicial precedents of criminal courts and provincial courts have considered that ayahuasca is not subject to the control regime of international treaties and that, therefore, its possession or sale is not criminally relevant, with some recent cases having resulted in acquittals and the return of the seized ayahuasca.

Thus, one of the latest court rulings, obtained by Francisco Azorín Ortega, the author of this appendix, states:

To recapitulate, at the international level it seems clear that, either in its plant presentation or as a preparation (paradigmatically decoction for oral ingestion, which is the case here), ayahuasca cannot be understood to be included in the 1971 Convention, even though DMT is; and therefore, as a decoction or in its plant presentation (the plants from which it is obtained), it is not subject to international control.

As a conclusion of this absence of specific mention at the national level and the lack of legal coverage in the 1971 Convention for its inclusion, we, therefore, understand that this preparation is not subject to special control in Spain, nor can it, therefore, be included in the definition of Article 368 of the Criminal Code.[24]

4.3 Pre-Trial Detention for False Positive Methamphetamine Tests

A person who was eventually acquitted for receiving a package with ayahuasca from Peru spent three months in prison because the substance showed a false positive for methamphetamine in the presumptive colorimetric test carried out by the police (something that usually happens with these plants). Therefore, until the substance was analyzed by a laboratory, with a confirmatory test, and until the corresponding appeals were filed because ayahuasca is not controlled, the investigated prisoner could not be released. Despite this, the antidrug prosecutor's office charged him with a crime against public health and asked for four years in prison.

There are also cases in which the investigating courts have ordered provisional imprisonment for the seizure of tobacco snuffs called rapé, sometimes containing DMT, which can show a false positive result for amphetamine or MDMA in the presumptive colorimetric tests carried out at customs. Even though a document from the Spanish Customs and Excise Department states that—even though almost all proceedings end in a file or acquittal and, normally, people who travel with suitcases loaded with ayahuasca from Colombia or Peru are no longer sent to provisional prison—controlled deliveries of ayahuasca should not be carried out, the truth is that as the appearance of these is that of a substance in greyish powder form that gives a false positive for MDMA, there have

---

24. Sentence from the Provincial Court (Audiencia Provincial) of Málaga (Sección 1ª) No. 86/2021 March 10.

been provisional incarcerations for such rapés. In other words, if 3 or 4 kilos of rapés are seized and thus produce a false positive result, it is easy to be sent to prison until the health department determines, in a confirmatory manner, the substance in question and its quantification, an injustice that confirms the deficiencies of the system and the lack of public resources and knowledge when it comes to the state exercising its greatest power, the punitive power, or what the Romans called *ultima ratio* or the ultimate "reason of state": criminal law. Pretrial detentions have been criticized multiple times by the renowned criminal justice lawyer Gerardo Landrove Díaz as "legalized injustice."

5. COUNTRIES THAT HAVE RECOGNIZED OR BANNED CERTAIN PLANTS WITH CONTROLLED MOLECULES AS PSYCHOTROPIC

5.1 Lack of Clarity in the Wording of International Conventions

As mentioned above, the legal interpretation of the international accounting of plants containing molecules controlled as psychotropic by the 1971 Convention has never been simple or peaceful and has always generated controversy.

All this controversy stems from the wording of the international conventions and their official commentaries.

Sánchez and Bouso (2015) state in a report:

> What does not seem to be so clear is whether, in order to continue allowing the traditional use of these psychoactive plants, a state party to the convention must formulate a reservation or not. Reading the text of the treaty, one would say yes. But the commentary introduces a statement that, in a way, creates a paradox concerning what the convention itself establishes: when it says that ". . . Continued tolerance of the use of the hallucinogenic substances mentioned at the 1971 Conference does not require the formulation of a reservation under paragraph 4 of Article 32 since, following the traditional way of dealing with this issue in the framework of international drug

control, the commentators consider that 'the inclusion in Schedule
I of the active ingredient of a substance does not mean that the substance itself is also included in the Schedule if it is a substance clearly
distinct from the substance which constitutes its active ingredient.'"

Therefore, there exists a disparity between the text of the convention and its official commentary signed by the U.N. Secretary-General.
This discrepancy was clarified by the INCB in the above-mentioned
reports of 2010 and 2012, which stated that these plants are not subject
to international control.[25]

5.2 Countries that Have Made Exceptions to International Conventions and Rulings Clarifying This Issue

Only Mexico, Peru, the United States, and Canada have indeed made
reservations to the 1971 international treaty to allow certain traditional
uses of these substances by native communities in the Amazon basin or
Indigenous reservations in the United States and Canada.[26]

In Chile, for example, a judgment was handed down in 2012
(Manto Wasi case) in which an ayahuasca ceremony had been infil-
trated by a police officer. It was considered that ayahuasca could not be
identified with DMT, controlled by the 1971 international convention
and Decree No. 867 of 2007 of the Andean country controlling DMT,
but that *P. viridis* and *B. cappi*, the individual plant components used
to prepare ayahuasca, could be. The ruling stated that ayahuasca did
not pose a danger to public health, and following the case, the director of public health requested that the Ministry of the Interior control
ayahuasca. The initiative did not go forward.[27]

France, however, does follow a prohibitionist model. In 1999, a

---

25. Sánchez C, Bouso JC. 2015. Ayahuasca: de la Amazonía a la aldea global
[Ayahuasca: from the Amazon to the global village]. Barcelona (Spain): International
Center for Ethnobotanical Education, Research, and Service. Spanish. Retrieved from
the Transnational Institute website.
26. Sánchez C, Bouso JC. 2015. (See full reference in note 25 of this appendix.)
27. Martín A, Muñoz J. 2019. (See full reference in note 11 of this appendix.)

controversy arose over a complaint by a mother of a member of a dai-mist group[28] who claimed that her son had lost touch with reality. The case resulted in a conviction by the Paris Court of First Instance on January 15, 2004. The ruling was appealed to the Paris Court of Appeal, which ruled on January 13, 2015, that, although ayahuasca has hallucino-genic effects, it can be distinguished from synthetic DMT, which is what is undoubtedly subject to the prohibition under French law. Furthermore, it was not possible to speak of a preparation in the technical and legal sense, as this would require the existence of a pure substance. As a result, the court ruled in favor of acquittal (Martín and Muñoz 2019). This pro-nouncement caused alarm among the authorities who, in order to avoid the situation highlighted in the ruling, decided to include all plants that are used or usually used in ayahuasca decoctions in the decree of April 20, 2005, thus prohibiting the uses of this plant in France (Martín and Muñoz 2019). Likewise, Italy banned ayahuasca in 2022.

5.3 Religious Uses and Cultural Heritage

In Brazil, a country with a strong "ayahuasca" culture, religious uses are recognized. Moreover, Brazil has not made a reservation to the 1971 Convention, and in 1985 the Ministry of Health included *B. cappi* and *P. viridis* as controlled substances. However, the "ayahuasca church," the União do Vegetal (UDV), fought a legal battle, which led to a study being carried out in communities that use ayahuasca in order to show that it had a significant positive effect (absence of alcoholism, lower infant mortality and malnutrition, crime rates close to zero, absence of violence, and the like). As a result of this report, the exclusion of plant species used in the preparation of ayahuasca was declared by Resolution No. 6 of February 4, 1986 (Martín and Muñoz 2019).

Subsequently, Resolution No. 1 of May 25, 2010, of CONAD

---

28. Santo Daime is a syncretic spiritual practice that blends elements of Christianity with South American Indigenous traditions and African influences. Originating in the Brazilian Amazon in the 1930s, it was founded by Raimundo Irineu Serra, known as Mestre Irineu. Central to the Santo Daime religion is the sacramental consumption of ayahuasca, a psychoactive brew traditionally used by Indigenous peoples for spiritual and healing purposes.

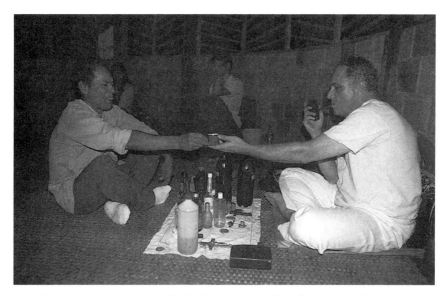

Ayahuasca ceremony at the Takiwasi Center (Peru). Image by Takiwasi.

(Council on Narcotic Drugs) ratified the legitimacy of the religious use of ayahuasca in one of the most detailed documents to date, regulating the uses of ayahuasca in religious practices, prohibiting its commercialization for profit, and emphasizing the avoidance of the offering in tourist packages (Martín and Muñoz 2019).

Peru, for its part, was the only country to make a distinction, under Article 32 of the 1971 Convention, regarding plants containing Schedule I psychotropic substances that have been traditionally used by certain small, clearly defined groups in religious ceremonies. This happened in 2008 when it declared ayahuasca a national cultural heritage. However, in contrast to Brazil, there is no detailed regulation, but rather a set of customs and practices.

Canada, the United States, and Colombia also allow religious uses of ayahuasca, and Canada and the United States also allow peyote cacti. In the Netherlands, religious uses of ayahuasca were allowed, but a Supreme Court ruling in 2019 changed the criteria and considered that the right to health prevails over religious freedom, declaring such use illegal.[29]

---

29. Ferrer I. 2019 Oct 2. El Supremo holandés prohíbe la importación de ayahuasca [Dutch Supreme Court bans the importation of ayahuasca]. El País (Madrid). Spanish.

5.4 Attempts to Ban a Multitude of Medicinal Plants by the Spanish State

In 2004, an attempt was made in Spain to ban by ministerial order a list of 197 plants that were considered toxic or dangerous by the government at the time. The case was appealed before the Audiencia Nacional, which, as well as the Supreme Court in its ruling of July 9, 2008, nullified the ministerial order of January 28, 2004, on the grounds of formal errors in the order. The prohibition of these plants was not attempted again in Spain, so they are not subject to national control, or, as we saw earlier, to international control.

5.5 The Case of Peyote: Countries that Made Exceptions and Those that Consider It Illegal

Regarding peyote, a report by the ICEERS Foundation states: "There are more than forty North American Indian tribes in many parts of the United States and Canada that use peyote as a religious sacrament."

The psychoactive alkaloid in peyote, mescaline, is a controlled substance under the 1971 Vienna Convention and is included in Schedule I. Its use, sale, and manufacture are therefore prohibited. However, the peyote plant is not included in the schedules of the conventions, and its regulation depends on the legislation of each country. Thus, in Canada, mescaline is in Schedule III, and peyote is explicitly exempted from regulation if it is not prepared for ingestion, whereas in Brazil, France, Italy, and other countries, peyote is considered illegal. Other countries, such as Spain, do not mention peyote in the lists of controlled plants, although this does not imply that the sale of peyote cannot be considered an illegal act.

In the case of U.S. legislation, the use of peyote is permitted only in ceremonial contexts for persons belonging to the Native American Church.

The Mexican government was one of the countries that, when adhering to the 1971 Convention and ratifying it on 20 February 1975, made an express reservation about its application, as there are certain Indigenous ethnic groups on its territory that traditionally use wild plants containing Schedule I psychotropic substances, including peyote. Within Mexican legislation, peyote cactus is not properly prohibited or regulated, as it is not included in any section of the General Health Law. Its use is permitted to the Huichols. Even so, peyote is considered an endangered plant, so, with exception of traditional use by Indigenous peoples, its collection is prohibited.[30]

6. DIFFERENCES BETWEEN CRIMINAL SIGNIFICANCE AND ADMINISTRATIVE REGULATION OF PLANTS CONTAINING MOLECULES CLASSIFIED AS PSYCHOTROPIC

To be fully aware of the legality surrounding these substances, it is necessary to differentiate between criminal and administrative legality. The truth is that the uses of ayahuasca and other plants are not authorized at the administrative level in almost any country in the world. Only certain religious uses exist, as we have pointed out in the previous section. In other words, plants with controlled substances cannot be sold as food or medicine, even if they are not expressly prohibited by international conventions or national laws transposing these conventions into national law.

6.1 Projections for Recognition of Medical Use of Psychedelics in the Short Term

This lack of administrative recognition will be short-lived. Clinical trials with psilocybin, MDMA, LSD, ibogaine, and DMT are well advanced, and it is expected that the use of these substances will soon be authorized by the U.S., Canadian, European, and worldwide drug agencies for the treatment of depression, PTSD, anxiety, addictions, and other medical conditions. Just recently, in July 2023, Australia authorized the medical use of psilocybin and MDMA by licensed psychiatrists for patients with depression and post-traumatic stress disorder, respectively, provided they meet specific requirements.

6.2 The Canadian Case

Even though they are controlled, due to scientific advances in the recognition of the therapeutic properties of these molecules, their advanced

---

30. Peyote: basic information. Retrieved from the ICEERS website.

clinical research stage into phases 2 and 3, the safety shown so far, and the need for new drugs in this field, given the delicate mental health situation exacerbated by the pandemic, the Canadian Health Agency (Health Canada) has just authorized doctors' access to psychedelic substances for mental health treatment.

In practice, this means that, in cases where other therapies have failed, are inadequate, or are unavailable in Canada, physicians are able, on behalf of patients with serious or life-threatening conditions, to apply for access to restricted medicines through Canada's Health Special Access Program (SAP).[31]

The proposed amendments are not intended to promote or encourage the early use of unapproved drugs, nor to circumvent well-established clinical trial or drug review and approval processes. However, these amendments could provide an additional potential option for physicians treating patients with serious or life-threatening conditions where other therapies have failed, are not suitable, or are not available.

As mentioned above, for the time being, ketamine or its isolate, esketamine, is the only substance that is currently fully administratively recognized. But very soon there will be more. Not only will cannabis be an administratively recognized medicine, but other, no less important substances (MDMA, psilocybin, DMT, and the like) are also knocking on the door to have their therapeutic properties recognized. One can already hear them: knock, knock!

In conclusion, the past and present research driven by people like Alexander Shulgin, Rick Doblin, Claudio Naranjo, David Nutt, Jordi Riba, Roland Griffiths, Amanda Fielding, José Carlos Bouso, Robin Carhart-Harris, the author of this book, and many others, will soon allow new substances, substances that have been unjustly stigmatized, demonized, abandoned, and banned for more than sixty years, to be authorized in order to deal more effectively with the pandemic of mental illness that plagues our societies.

---

31. Canada Gazette, Part I, Volume 154, No. 50: Government Notices. 2020 Dec 12.

7. HISTORICAL, ECOLOGICAL, AND CULTURAL REASONS WHY PLANTS WITH MOLECULES CLASSIFIED AS PSYCHOTROPIC WERE NOT BANNED

7.1 Historical and Cultural Reasons

The historical, ecological, and cultural reasons for this choice are varied, but we could say that plants containing the alkaloid dimethyltryptamine (DMT) and mushrooms containing psilocybin are very numerous and are found all over the world. This means that legislators would have to control substances that could grow naturally in any field or garden patch.

One of the most important books ever written on psychedelics, *TiHKAL*, authored by two of the world's most influential people in the study of psychedelics, Alexander and Ann Shulgin,[32] contains a chapter titled "DMT Is Everywhere."

The chapter "Botany of Tryptamines" can be found within the third part of the book and at its beginning, we can read the following:

What is at the top of the pyramid? N,N-dimethyltryptamine, or DMT, of course. I think this is the right time to talk about the substance and the Drug Law, as 1966 is an interesting time when both stories converge. Manske first synthesised DMT in 1931. It was then independently isolated from two different plants: in 1946 by Goncalves de Lima (from *Mimosa hostilis*) and in 1955 by Fish, Johnson, and Horning (from *Piptadenia peregrina*). In 1956 Szára reported its activity in humans as a synthetic entity. The first legal restrictions on its research came in 1966 in response to the growing popularity it gained through the literature of Burroughs, Metzner, Leary, and others in the early 1960s; and in 1976, Christian noted its involvement as a component of the healthy human brain (and perhaps as a neurotransmitter).

The year 1965 marked the beginning of the use of initials, both as to substance and organisation names, in Federal Law Enforcement.

---

32. Shulgin Alexander, Shulgin Ann. 1997. TiHKAL: the continuation. Berkeley (CA): Transform Press.

It was then that, largely motivated by the psychedelic hippie movement of the younger generation at the time, the Drug Abuse Control amendments were passed and came into force. This led to the founding of the BDAC (Bureau of Drug Abuse Control), which became part of the FDA. These amendments were drafted to try to control non-narcotic substances (so-called dangerous substances) such as DMT, LSD, DET, ibogaine, bufotenine, DOM, MDA, MDMA, and TMA. BDAC was an agency that acted in parallel, but not in contact, with the already existing FBN (Federal Bureau of Narcotics), which was exclusively dedicated to the control of the three known narcotic substances: heroin, cocaine, and marijuana. . . .

Therefore, the origin of the control of DMT as a pure substance comes from factors such as in synthesized onion, in both its pure and crystallized form, given it was synthesized even before it was discovered within countless plants, as well as to the fact that it is even found in the human brain, something that should not be so surprising given its similarity to the serotonin molecule and hence its metabolic proximity.

7.2 Ecological Reasons

A little further on, Shulgin and Shulgin (1997) continue: "The answer to the second question is that DMT is simply almost everywhere you look. It is in this flower here, in that tree there, and in those animals further away."

The book's chapter is divided into sections to indicate where DMT can be found: marine world (*S. ehina*, *S. auria*, etc.); toads (*Bufo*); herbs (birdseed or *Phalaris* species, etc.); legumes (*Acacia*, *Mimosa*, Illinois flower, *Sophora secundiflora* seed or mescal bean, etc.); *Psychotria* (*P. viridis*); limes, lemons, and Angostura bitters (*Zanthoxylum arborescens* and *Z. procerum*) (Shulgin and Shulgin 1997).

Different species of psilocybe mushrooms also grow wild around the world, as can be seen in various books. Many sources can be consulted to accredit the large number of mushrooms containing molecules that are controlled under international law (psilocin and psilocybin), but some notable ones are the following: *Psilocybin*

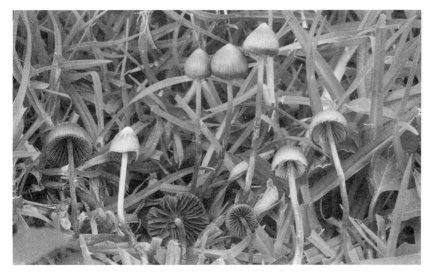

Psilocybe mexicana photographed in Veracruz, Mexico.
Image by Alan Rockefeller.

Mushrooms of the World,[33] *Psilocibes (The Mushrooms)*,[34] *Teonanácatl*,[35] and *Pharmacotheon*.[36] Almost all varieties of psilocybin mushrooms discovered up to the time of publication can be consulted here.

In the book *Psilocibes*, we find chapter four, authored by Oscar Parés, which lists some of the existing varieties of mushrooms that contain psilocybin: *cubensis*, *Panaeolus/Copelandia cynescens*, and *Panaeolus/Copelandia tropicalis*.

The author states:

There is a third grouping of psilocybin fungi that is worth considering. It is not distinguished from the previous two by its genetic family but by its form or presentation. Called truffle (Latin: *sclerotium*, plural: *sclerotia*), it is a hardened compact mass of mycelium containing

33. Stamets P. 1996. Psilocybin mushrooms of the world: an identification guide. Berkeley (CA): Ten Speed Press.
34. Bouso JC, editor. 2013. Psilocibes: the mushrooms. Motril (Spain): Ultraradio.
35. Ott J, Bigwood J, Wasson G, Belmonte D, Hoffmann A, Weil A, Evans R. 1985. Teonanácatl: hongos alucinógenos de Europa y América del Norte [Teonanácatl (flesh of the gods): hallucinogenic mushrooms of Europe and North America]. Madrid: Swan. Spanish.
36. Ott J. 1996. Pharmacotheon. Barcelona (Spain): La Liebre de Marzo.

psilocybin. It is produced when the environmental conditions are not favourable for the flower, or reproductive apparatus (read: the fungus) to sprout from the long underground mycelium. Under this heading, we would include the most widespread *Psilocybe tampanensis*, but sclerotia of *Psilocybe mexicana* and *Psilocybe atlantis* are also commercially available.

7.2.1 Psilocybe Fungi Found on the Iberian Peninsula

Following the quotation in the previous section:

> *Psilocybe cyanescens* and *Copelandia cyanescens* are also known to have been found in open fields on the Iberian Peninsula. . . .
>
> We now turn to two other psilocybe fungi of special interest that occur in the Iberian context. The first of these is *Psilocybe hispanica*. This fungus was discovered in the Huesca Pyrenees.
>
> In Galicia, we find the *Psilocybe gallaeciae*, which according to Guzmán, one of the most prestigious mycologists in the world, belongs to the variety *P. mexicana*. There are indications that two other mushrooms with psilocybin content can be found in Catalonia: *Psilocybe subbalteatus* and *Panaelus cyanescens*.

The book we have just quoted also contains a chapter titled "Visionary Fungi" in the Iberian Peninsula, written by Ignacio Seral Bozal.

To get an idea of the number of psychoactive mushrooms that are not legally controlled and exist in the Iberian Peninsula, we will cite the different sections into which this chapter is divided such as we previously did with the *TiHKAL* chapter.

- *Amanita muscaria*.[37] Species: *A. phantherina* and *A. gemmata*.
- Genus *Panaeolus*. Species: *P. cyanescens*.
- Genus *Pluteus*. Species: *P. salicinus* and *P. antricapillus*.
- Genus *Inocybe*. Species: *I. aemacta*, *I. corydalina*, *I. coelestium*, and *I. aeruginascens*.

---

37. Psychoactive but not psychedelic mushroom.

- Genus *Gymnopilus*. Species: *G. spectabilis*.
- Genus *Psilocybe*. Species: *P. hispanicae*, *P. galicae*, *P. cyanescens*, and *P. semilanceata*.

As we can see, the argument put forward to defend the noncontrol of plants with DMT content is also applicable in the case of psilocybe mushrooms. There are many genera and species of psychoactive mushrooms in the world. Some of them, such as *A. muscaria*, do not even contain controlled molecules. Ibotenic acid and muscimol (the psychoactive ingredients of this species) are not subject to international control; therefore, in this case, it would not even raise doubts regarding varieties of mushrooms that contain controlled molecules that we are trying to resolve. Despite this lack of regulation, the consumption of this mushroom does not produce classic psychedelic effects and actually poses far more health risks than any other psilocybin-containing fungal species.

Bearing this in mind, in the case of a hypothetical control of these mushrooms, one could present the exception of the international convention that states that if the organism grows wild in that territory and there is a traditional use, reservations to the convention could be accepted.

Mescaline-containing cacti are also present not only in American countries but also in Spain and other southern European countries.

7.3 Reasons Given in the 2014 TNI Report

To understand a little more about how these international conventions were put together, let us quote a paragraph from a TNI report (Transnational Institute 2014):

> The problem regarding how to deal with the traditional uses of certain plants arose again at the 1971 Conference, especially concerning psilocybin-containing mushrooms and the mescaline-containing peyote cactus, both hallucinogenic substances listed in the 1971 Convention schedules. Then, as of now, mushrooms and peyote were used in religious and healing ceremonies by Mexican and North American Indigenous groups. Unlike the position they took during the 1961 negotiations, this time the US authorities

accepted the "consensus that it is not worth trying to impose control measures on biological substances from which psychotropic substances can be obtained . . . North American Indians in the United States and Mexico use peyote in religious rites and the misuse of this substance is considered sacrilege." By excluding plants from which alkaloids could be extracted from the scheduled lists, the 1971 Convention deviated, with good reason, from the prevailing zero-tolerance rule that had been applied in the Single Convention [on Narcotic Drugs]. The very concept of "psychotropic substances" was a distortion of the logic underpinning the control framework, as the term lacks scientific credentials and was originally invented, in effect, as an excuse to avoid the much stricter controls of the Single Convention being applied to the wide range of psychoactive, mostly synthetic, drugs included in the 1971 Convention.[38]

7.4 Conclusion

There may be several reasons as to why no plants are controlled under the 1971 Convention on Psychotropic Substances. One of the most likely reasons is the fact that if all plants containing any active substances categorized as a psychotropic were to be banned, a large part of the world's flora would be illegal. Given that in some other instances some plants are indeed controlled, it may also be that the conventions understand that it is not desirable to control plants that are not considered extremely dangerous. After all, unlike controlled plants such as the opium poppy or the coca plant, which could kill in high doses, psychedelic plant sources rarely pose a direct risk to physical health.

In conclusion, it seems that solid arguments exist such as mental health, risk and harm reduction, and what is known as the "management of risks and pleasures," and not only on a scientific but also on a historical, legal, cultural, and ecological level. These arguments can and should be taken into account by both the readers and public authorities when, with the greatest legal guarantees, facilitating access to psychedelic therapy.

---

38. Henman A, Metaal P. 2014. Hora de abrir los ojos [It's time to open our eyes]. Amsterdam (The Netherlands): Transnational Institute. Spanish.

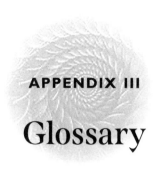

Glossary

ADDICTION: Pathological search for reward or relief through the use of a substance or other actions. Usually associated with negative consequences and an inability to control behavior, as well as a dysfunctional emotional response. As for psychoactive substances, there is less and less talk of addiction and *more of a substance use disorder.*

ALKALOIDS: Secondary plant metabolites, usually synthesized from amino acids, which have in common their water solubility at acidic pH and their solubility in organic solvents at alkaline pH. True alkaloids are derived from an amino acid and are therefore nitrogenous. All those with the amine or imine functional group are basic. Many psychoactive substances are alkaloids.

BASELINE STATE: State of sobriety and normal consciousness that is considered the beginning or end of the effects of a psychoactive drug.

BOMB: Psychoactive substance, in a certain quantity and wrapped in a cigarette paper, for oral consumption, as a capsule.

BRAIN-DERIVED NEUROTROPHIC FACTOR (BDNF): Protein that acts as a growth factor for neuronal tissue. Data have accumulated showing that BDNF has an important role in the physiological processes underlying neuroplasticity and development of the nervous system.

CRIMINAL SIGNIFICANCE: When an alleged offense is covered by an article of the criminal code of a given state and the consequence is a legal measure consisting of a custodial sentence, a financial penalty, or the deprivation of a fundamental right, such as disqualification from holding public office, disqualification from participating in elections, or disqualification from association with the victim.

There are also security measures consisting of the internment of persons who are not criminally liable, such as those who have committed the offense because of a psychiatric illness.

DAIMISTA: Parishioner of the Church of Santo Daime (ayahuasca church).

DEA: Drug Enforcement Administration. It is the agency of the U.S. Department of Justice dedicated to combating the smuggling and use of illegal drugs in the United States, as well as money laundering. Although it shares jurisdiction with the FBI, domestically, along with U.S. Immigration and Customs Enforcement and U.S. Customs and Border Protection, it is the sole agency responsible for coordinating and prosecuting antidrug investigations abroad.

DEFAULT MODE NETWORK (DMN): Network of interacting brain regions that is active when a person is not engaged in activities nor focused on the outside world. It is considered a high-hierarchy network that influences and filters lower-hierarchy networks, such as sensory ones, and its appeasement under the effects of psychedelics is related to the experience of ego dissolution or "ego death."

DESIGNER DRUG: Engineering in the synthesis of new drugs whose mission is to create substances that mimic other substances under international or national control. The classic example of a designer drug would be fentanyl, which mimics controlled opiates. And the paradigm of a psychedelic designer drug would be 2CB, synthesized by A. Shulgin in 1974 in an attempt to find a molecule similar to mescaline. Terms such as NPS (new psychoactive substance) or RC (research chemicals) are also used to define these when they are very new and not yet internationally controlled.

DETOXIFICATION TREATMENT: A measure imposed by a court as a substitute for a prison sentence for drug-related offenses. The convicted person must complete the treatment under the warning that, if they fail to attend the appointments, or fail to complete the treatment, the benefit of the suspended sentence will be revoked.

DRUG OR PSYCHOACTIVE SUBSTANCE: Any chemical substance that, upon entering the body via any route (buccal, nasal, oral, intravenous, or others by which the substance can be absorbed), exerts a direct effect on the central nervous system through neuroreceptors and causes specific changes in its functions. These substances are capable of inhibiting pain, modifying mood or emotions, or altering perceptions. Psychoactive substances have been used in all kinds of medical, ritual, religious, and recreational contexts (examples are opium, alcohol, nicotine, caffeine, cocaine, and morphine).

EUROPEAN UNION DRUGS AGENCY (EUDA): A European public agency set up to monitor and publish reports on the prevalence of drug use in the states of the European Union and to assess and advise on drug policy.

FEDERAL LAWS: Laws passed in the U.S. Congress. They differ from the laws of individual states in that they affect all American citizens and can only deal with certain very important competencies attributed by the U.S. Constitution to the U.S. Congress, located on Capitol Hill in Washington, DC. The FBI (Federal Bureau of Investigation) is responsible for investigating offenses covered by and punishable under federal law.

HARM REDUCTION: Compendium of tools and strategies that seek to reduce the harm associated with an activity, such as the use of psychoactive substances, in populations in which that activity is already causing harm. In English, there is no formal differentiation between risk reduction and harm reduction, and both are considered to be included in the definition of harm reduction.

ICEERS FOUNDATION: A nonprofit foundation based in the Netherlands and Spain dedicated to the research of applications of plants containing psychoactive molecules, controlled or not, for the treatment of different diseases, as well as to the protection of the cultures that use them in a traditional way. They have ECOSOC status at the United Nations Commission on Narcotic Drugs.

INTEGRATION: Process after a psychedelic experience in which the content that has emerged is processed and worked on from a psychotherapeutic perspective, emphasizing applying the abstract to real life. It is considered one of the most important parts of psychedelic-assisted psychotherapy or any other therapeutic work with psychedelics.

INTERNATIONAL CONVENTION ON PSYCHOTROPIC SUBSTANCES:
Together with the 1961 Single Convention on Narcotic Drugs and the 1988 United Nations Convention against Illicit Traffic in Narcotic Drugs and Psychotropic Substances, the 1971 Convention forms the current international drug control system. It was prompted by the rise in the use of hallucinogenic or psychedelic drugs and to control nonnarcotic substances, such as those included in the 1961 Convention.

INTERNATIONAL NARCOTICS CONTROL BOARD, INCB (NCBI):
An independent, quasi-judicial body of experts established under the 1961 Single Convention on Narcotic Drugs by the merger of two bodies, namely the Central Standing Committee on Narcotic Drugs, established under the 1925 International Opium Convention, and the Narcotics Control Bureau, established under the 1931 Convention for Limiting the Manufacture and Regulating the Distribution of Narcotic Drugs. INCB consists of thirteen members, each elected to serve for a term of five years by the Economic and Social Council.

JURISPRUDENCE: Doctrine established repeatedly by the Supreme Court or the Constitutional Court when interpreting the constitution and its laws.

LEGISLATION: A set of rules and laws that regulate the relations between people in a country or a particular sector. Legislation makes it possible to organize a given sector and a country as a whole.

MAPS (MULTIDISCIPLINARY ASSOCIATION FOR PSYCHEDELIC STUDIES): A nonprofit organization founded in 1984 by Rick Doblin to research the medical and cultural uses of psychedelic substances.

MICRODOSING: Refers to the practice of using doses of psychedelics, such as LSD or psychoactive mushrooms, but below the minimum threshold to notice their psychoactive effects. People who microdose psychedelics report using them as a form of therapy and to increase creativity and intellectual performance. Given the recentness of the practice and the low number of studies, it has not been possible to scientifically verify the claims about the positive or negative impacts of this practice in the short, medium, and long term. From the psychedelic community, the use of microdosing has been criticized for using psychedelics to turn a "counterculture sacrament" into one more way to engage in productivity and the consumer society. It has also been suggested that continuous use could increase the risk of certain heart conditions in its users predisposed to heart disease.

MINISTERIAL ORDER: A legal instrument of Spanish law that is not strictly speaking a law, decree, or regulation, and which serves, in this case, to include substances in one or another list of the different national drug laws that transpose international conventions into domestic law.

MKULTRA: Secret CIA project looking for military and espionage uses for various psychoactive substances (including psychedelics) and other techniques. During its years of operation (1953–1973), macabre secret experiments were carried out on volunteers or chosen people without their knowledge or consent, some of which ended in death.

MONOAMINE OXIDASE INHIBITOR (MAOI): Substance that inhibits the activity of monoamine oxidase enzymes; closely related to the degradation of neurotransmitters and psychoactive substances. They were the first antidepressants on the market.

MYSTICAL EXPERIENCE: Very personal introspective experience where some kind of universal unity or transcendence of time and space is described. They can occur at high doses of psychedelics, and are often associated with better long-term therapeutic outcome, so they are now often sought in psychedelic-assisted psychotherapy settings.

NARCOTIC SUBSTANCES: These are the substances included in the 1971 Convention on Psychotropic Substances. This is a legal or juridical term that includes those substances in Schedules I and II of the 1961 Convention on Narcotic Drugs. Moreover, many of those included in this book could not be defined as narcotic drugs, but cannabis would also be defined as hallucinogenic, or semipsychedelic. And cocaine, which is not a narcotic in a strict sense, can be considered as a local anesthetic with stimulant properties.

NEURON: Main component cell of the nervous system. Its mission is to receive, process, and transmit nerve impulses that come from other neurons through chemical signals (neurotransmitters) or in the form of electrical impulses. The connection between neurons or with other types of cells is called a synapse.

NEUROPHARMACOLOGY: Study of how drugs affect cell function in the nervous system and the neural mechanisms that influence behavior.

NEUROPLASTICITY: Ability of the neural networks of the brain (and the neurons that make them up) to modify their shape and connections (synapses) to adapt to changes in the environment or new requirements, either through learning or other adaptations.

NEURORECEPTOR OR NEUROTRANSMITTER RECEPTOR: Protein complexes located in the cell membranes of neurons and that act as a lock in a door, allowing the interaction of certain substances (neurotransmitters) with the mechanisms of cellular metabolism as well as chemical communication between cells and the synapse process.

NEUROSCIENCE: Field of science that studies the nervous system and all its aspects, such as its structure, function, development, biochemistry, pharmacology, and pathology and how its different elements interact, giving rise to the biological bases of cognition and behavior.

NEUROTRANSMITTER: Molecule responsible for transmitting signals from one neuron to the next, linked by a synapse. The neurotransmitter is released at the tip of the presynaptic neuron during nerve impulse propagation, crosses the synaptic gap, and acts by changing the action potential in the next neuron, called postsynaptic.

ONEIRONAUT: Explorer of altered states of consciousness produced during sleep and lucid dreaming.

PLACEBO: Pharmacologically inert substance that is administered to a patient as if it were a medicine in order to compare its effect with that of a real drug, and thus rule out the effects produced by simple suggestion or expectancy.

POST-TRAUMATIC STRESS DISORDER (PTSD): Mental disorder classified within the group of those related to traumas and stress factors. It is characterized by the appearance of specific symptoms after exposure to a stressful event, extremely traumatic, of an extraordinarily threatening or catastrophic nature for the individual, even when the threat no longer exists.

PRESUMPTIVE COLOR TEST: A field test performed by the police to provide a quick indication that a particular substance may be classified as a narcotic or psychotropic substance. It differs from confirmatory tests in that, in presumptive tests, there is a possibility of false positives and negatives, and it is not possible to quantify the purity of the substance seized and, therefore, whether it exceeds the minimum psychoactive dose, or whether it is a toxic dose. Examples of a presumptive test: Duquenois or Marquis.

PROPORTIONALITY TEST: Legal doctrine for the interpretation of conflicting fundamental rights in a legal relationship, whether these concern two fundamental rights of the individual, or a right of the individual as opposed to collective legal goods, such as public health or collective security.

PSYCHEDELIC: Substance whose main action is to alter the cognition, emotion, and perception of the mind, giving rise to nonordinary perceptions. The term is derived from the Greek words ψυχή (psyche, "mind") and δηλείν (dileín, "to manifest"), which can be translated as "manifestation of the mind/soul." Normally, this effect is produced by action on the serotonin 5-HT2a neuroreceptor. Psychedelic drugs are also known by the names of hallucinogenic drugs, entheogenic drugs, visionary drugs, power drugs, psychodysleptics, psychotomimetics, and eidetics. Each of these names is associated with a particular worldview, is not always appropriate in all contexts, and none fully describes the psychophysiological effects.

PSYCHONAUTICS/PSYCHONAUT: From the Greek ψυχή (psyche, "mind") and ναύτης (naútes, "sailor or navigator"); refers to the methodology for describing and explaining the subjective effects of alternate states of consciousness, including states induced by mind-altering substances or meditation. The researcher voluntarily plunges into an altered state through these techniques to explore human experience and existence.

PSYCHOTROPIC SUBSTANCES: Those included in the 1971 Convention on Psychotropic Substances. As with narcotic drugs, this is a legal term for such substances that can be classified as stimulants (amphetamine) or hallucinogens (LSD).

REGULATION: A rule that develops the content of a law.

REMISSION: Reduction of symptoms associated with a mental disorder. Remission can be partial or complete. In mental health, the word "cure" is not often used.

RESERVATION TO AN INTERNATIONAL TREATY: A unilateral act by which a State or an international organization expresses its intention to exclude or modify an obligation arising from an international treaty.

RISK: Probability of a negative event or damage occurring. However, it does not necessarily imply that it will occur. For example, leaning over a ledge means exposing yourself to a risk of falling, but it does not necessarily imply that it will happen (and therefore cause damage).

RISK REDUCTION: Compendium of tools and strategies that seek to reduce the risks associated with an activity that can be dangerous, such as the consumption of psychoactive substances, when you do not want to give up said activity. Risk reduction in the use of psychoactive substances is applied to a population that has not yet suffered harm from its use and is to prevent its occurrence. In English, there is no formal differentiation between risk reduction and harm reduction, and both are considered to be included in the definition of harm reduction.

SECOND SUMMER OF LOVE: A social phenomenon between 1988 and 1989 in the United Kingdom during which acid house music developed, providing the soundtrack for the emergence of the rave culture, a synergistic combination of a drug (namely ecstasy, where it was also known as "E") together with another way of understanding music recreationally through group dance.

SINGLE CONVENTION ON NARCOTIC DRUGS: The international treaty signed on March 30, 1961, in New York, which forms the international legal framework for drug control. The convention defined narcotic drugs as "any of the substances in Schedules I and II, natural or synthetic," and recognizes in its preamble that the medical use of narcotic drugs is indispensable for the relief of pain and that State signatories to the treaty should take "the necessary measures to ensure the availability of narcotic drugs for such purposes."

SYNAPSE: Zone of approximation between two neurons, like a connector, through which chemical signals (neurotransmitters) are sent. It allows neuronal signals to spread. Depending on the type of element that is transmitted between neurons, we can find chemical synapses (majority in our body) and electrical synapses.

TOLERANCE: Gradual process of physiological adaptation that occurs as a result of continued exposure or administration to a substance, and which will cause the subject to be less sensitive to it. Thus, the usual dose of the substance produces progressively fewer effects, so higher doses are needed to produce them.

TRIPSITTER: Sober person accompanying someone who is having a psychedelic experience. Their job is to take care of the person's safety and help them manage the experience if they need it.

UNIÃO DO VEGETAL (UDV): Together with Santo Daime, another of the biggest ayahuasca churches in the world.

UNITED NATIONS COMMISSION ON NARCOTIC DRUGS (CND): Established by the Economic and Social Council (ECOSOC) of the United Nations by Resolution 9 of February 17, 1946, as the governing body of international drug control treaties. It is a functional commission of the ECOSOC. The CND meets annually in Vienna, Austria, to examine and adopt a series of decisions and resolutions related to the implementation of drug treaties and policies about narcotic drugs and psychotropic substances.

WAR ON DRUGS: A policy promoted by the U.S. government aimed at the prosecution of the production, trade, and consumption of certain psychoactive substances. The term was popularized by the media shortly after a press conference held on June 18, 1971, by U.S. President Richard Nixon.

Index

Page numbers in *italics* indicate illustrations

1P-LSD, 33–37
2-FDCK, 30–33
2M2B, 21–23
5-HT2a receptors, 99–100, 111–12
5-MeO-DMT, 33–37, 164–67,
    235
6-APB, 26–30
25i-NBOMe, 33–37

acetylcholine, *6–7*
acid test, 53
activism, 228–29
addictions, 134–40
ADHD, 18–19, *18*
Adley, Mark, 17
administration routes, 118, 205–6
adulteration, 201–5
Africa, 254
alcohol, 20–23
Alcoholics Anonymous, 45–47
Alpert, Richard, 53–54
alpha-PVP, 18
amphetamines, 18
antidepressants, 74
anxiety, 125–34

anxiolytics, 215
apples, 215
Argentina, 249
Asia, 254
axons, *3–5*
ayahuasca, *pl.17*, 158–64, *160*, *161*,
    255, *256*
ayahuasca church, 260

bad trips, 32, 157, 163, 190–91,
    213–16
bans against psychedelics, 67–70
Barbanoj, Manel, 77
barbiturates, 20–23
Beckley Foundation, 75, 226
behavior change, 142
Bell, Kristen, 90
benzodiazepines, 20–23, 74, 215
Berkeley Center for the Science of
    Psychedelics (BCSP), 91
Betts, Leah, 246
Bicycle Day, 42–43, 91
bipolar disorder, 209
black cohosh, 207
Blewett, Duncan, 52

Bluelight, 75–76
bodyweight, 200
books, 232–33
Bouso, José Carlos, 78, 264
Bozal, Ignacio Seral, 268–69
brain, 1–3, *2*
    hierarchical predictive coding and,
        101–5
    how psychedelics affect function,
        pl.10, *pl.11*, 105–8, *106*, *108*
Brazil, 260–61, *262*
breathing exercises, 214
Brotherhood of Eternal Love, 62
Bufo alvarius, 164–65, 235
buprenorphine, 23–24
Burning Man, 90–91, *92*
Burroughs, William, 53

cactus, 167–73
caffeine, 18–19, 203
Canada, 259–60, *262*, 263–64
cancer patients, 49–50, 132–233
cannabinoids, 24–26
cannabis, *pl.25*, 207–8
Cannabiscafe, 75–76
Carcillo, Daniel, 90
cardiovascular risks, 182
Carhart-Harris, Robin, *pl.3*, 90,
        100–101, 114–15, 264
cathinones, 204
central nervous system (CNS), 1–3, *2*
changa, 160
Chile, 259–60
CIA, 50
cocaine, 18
codeine, 23–24
cognitive alterations, 149, 170

Cohen, Sidney, 47, 49–50
Colombia, 248–49, 257–58
Colorado, 241–43
combinations, 207–8
Compass Pathways, 84
conflict resolution, 142–43
consciousness, 109–10
Convention on Psychotropic
        Substances, 269–70
couples therapy, 142–43
COVID-19, 74, 140–41
creativity, 56, 94–96
Crick, Francis, 56
cultural heritage, 260–61
current affairs, 230
Cyrus, Miley, 90

dancing, 185
death, fear of, 49–50
decriminalization, 216, 241–43
default mode network (DMN),
        100–101, 107–8, 109, 112–14
dehydration, 182
delirium tremens, 22, 45
Delysid, *50*, 61, 153
dendrites, 3–4, *3*
depressants, 20–23
depression, 125–34
Díaz, Gerardo Landrove, 258
dilution, 202
dissociatives, 30–33
DMT, *pl.16*, 33–37, 158–64, *158*
Doblin, Rick, 66–67, 90, 97, 247, 264
documentaries, 230–31
doors of perception, 105
dopamine, 5, *6–7*, 8
dosage, 198–201

drug analysis, 196, 228
Drug Enforcement Administration,
    U.S. (DEA), 65, 70, 237
DrugsData, 200, 205
Drugs-Forum, 75–76
Drugs Wheel, The, *pl.6, pl.7*, 17
"Drugs World," 16–17
drug testing, 184

echinacea, 207
ecstasy. *See* MDMA
ego death, 109–10
Ellis, Havelock, 40
emergencies, 213–16
empathogens, 26–30. *See also*
    entactogens
Energy Control, 200, 205
entactogens, 26–30. *See also*
    empathogens
Erowid, 75–76
esketamine, 30–31, 83–84, 126,
    133–34, 187–88
European Medicines Agency (EMA),
    217–24
European Parliament, 217–24
evasion, 193

Fadiman, James, 55–56, 90, 143–45
Feilding, Amanda, 90
fentanyl, 23–24, 204
Ferriss, Tim, 90, 94
festivals, 90–91
Feynman, Richard, 56
flashbacks, 191
follow-up, 118–19
Food and Drug Administration
    (FDA), 56–57

forums, 229
Foucault, Michel, 56
Fox, Megan, 90
France, 253, 259–60, 262
frequency of consumption, 198–201
Friston, Karl, 100–101
fun, 193

GABA, *6–7*
gender differences, 200
GHB, 16, 21–23
ginkgo biloba, 207
Ginsberg, Allen, 53
Global Drug Survey, 91
glutamate, *6–7*
God molecule, 164, 166
Golden Gate Park, 61
Gouzoulis-Mayfrank, Euphrosyne, 77
Grant, Cary, 52, 236
grape seed extract, 215
green out, 26
Greer, George, 69
Grey, Alex, 90, 161
Griffiths, Roland, 78–79, 90
Grob, Charles, 77
Grof, Paul, 66
Grof, Stanislav, 90

hallucinogen persistent perception
    disorder (HPPD), 191
haloperidol, 215
hangovers, 183
hard drugs, 15
harm reduction, 192–97, *193, 195,*
    197. See also risks
    administration routes, 205–6
    bad trips, 213–16

classification of drugs, 220
dosage, frequency, and tolerance, 198–201
graphs of, *pl.26*, *pl.27*
mixtures and combinations, 207–8
purity and adulteration, 201–5
resources, 225–26, 227–28
set and setting, 208–13
Harris, Sam, 90
hawthorn, 215
Heffter, Arthur, 39, *39*
Heffter Research Institute, 75
Heim, Roger, 51
heroin, 23–24
hierarchical predictive coding, 101–5
hippies, 95–96
history of psychedelics
    alcoholism and, 45–47
    post-LSD, 40–63
    pre-LSD, 38–40
Hoffer, Abram, 44, 46, 57
Hofmann, Albert, 40–43, 47, 55, 71, 79–80, *80*
hollow mask illusion, 103–5, *104*
hormones, 5
Hubbard, Alfred, 46–47, 52
Huxley, Aldous, 47–48, *48*
hydration, 211
hypericum, 207
hyperthermia, 183
hyponatremia, 183

Iberian Peninsula, 268–69
ibogaine, *pl.20*, *pl.21*, 173–77, *174*, *175*
ICEERS, 75, 78

Illinois, 243
Imperial College London, 86, *86*, 114–15
Indocybin, 52
industry, rise of, 93–97
inhalation, 206
INSIGHT, 83, *83*
integration, 118
intentions, 117, 210
International Convention on Psychotropic Substances, 237
International Narcotics Control Board (INCB), 255, 256
internet, 75–76
intravenous administration, 206
Italy, 253, 260, 262

Jobs, Steve, 56, 93–94, *95*
Johns Hopkins University, 75
Johnson, Matthew, 90
Jünger, Ernst, 47

Kafkalides, Athanasios, 69
kale, 215
Kast, Erik, 48–49
kava, 207
Kennedy, John F., 55
Kennedy, Robert, 52, 60
Kesey, Ken, 53, 236
ketamine, *pl.24*, 30–33
    about, 186–91, *188*
    legal status of, 238–41
    research and, 78
khat, 255
Kleiman, Mark, 238
Kleinman, Merrie, 63

Klüver, Heinrich, 40
Köllisch, Anton, 63

Latin America, 248–49
Leary, Timothy, 53–55, *54*, 61, 236
Lee, Ben, 90
legal status of psychedelics, 89
  control of psychotropic plants,
    254–58
  criminal significance and
    administrative regulation,
    263–64
  introduction to, 234–41
  penalties for trafficking and use,
    244–54
  reasons for not banning, 265–70
  resources for information, 233
Lilly, John C., 56
lithium, 207
lock and key analogy, 9–10, *9*
LSD, 33–37, 139–40
  about, 153–57
  adulterants and, 204
  bans against psychedelics, 60–63
  Hofmann and, 40–43
  pictured, *pl.8, pl.15*

magnesium, 215
Maine, 243
Malleson, Nicolas, 57
manuals, 231
MAOIs, 159–60, 163
Massachusetts, 243
McCandless, David, 16–17
McCartney, Paul, 90
m-CPP, 203
MDA, 26–30

MDMA, *pl.22, pl.23*, 26–30, 63–67,
    119–25, 177–86, *179, 181*,
    223–24
  common adulterants and, 203–4
  research and, 78, 84–86
MDMC, 27
MDPV, 18
mebroqualone, 21–23
mental illness, 36–37, 76–77,
    112–15
Merry Pranksters, The, 53, *53*
mescaline, 33–37, 39–40, 167–73,
    169, 170, 262–63
methadone, 23–24
methamphetamines, 18, 257–58
Metzner, Ralph, 53–54
Mexico, 248–49, 259–60
Michigan, 243
microdosing, 56, 94–96, 143–45,
    221–22
Middle East, 254
milk thistle, 215
Millbrook, 54–55
Minnesota, 243
Mitchell, Weir, 40
mixtures, 207–8
MKUltra, 50, 63
morphine, 23–24
Morris, Hamilton, 90
Mullis, Kary, 56
Multidisciplinary Association for the
    Study of Psychedelics (MAPS),
    66–67, *68*, 75, 226
music, 212
Musk, Elon, 94
MXE, 30–33
mystical experiences, 110, 115

N2O, 30–33
naloxone, 24
Naranjo, Claudio, 264
National Institute of Mental Health,
    U.S. (NIMH), 57–58
Native American Church, 262–63
Netherlands, 252, 261
neurogenerative diseases, 140–41
neurons, *pl.2*, 3–9, *3*
neuropharmacology, 9–10
neuroreceptors, 3–10, 98–100
neurorehabilitation, 140–41
neurotoxicity, 183–84
neurotransmitters, 3–10
new psychoactive substances (NPS),
    204–5, 235
news, 230
NGO Espolea, 16–17
Nichols, David E., 63–64, 90
nicotine, 18
nitrous oxide, 30–33
Nixon, Richard, 61, 62–63, 237
nootropics, 19
norepinephrine, *6–7*
nourishment, 211, 214–15
Nutt, David, 90

Odom, Lamar, 90
omega-3 fatty acids, 215
opioids, 23–24, 207
optimism, 218
oral administration, 206
Oregon, 242–43
Ortega, Francisco Azorín,
    256–57
Osmond, Humphry, 44–45,
    46, 52

Paltrow, Gwyneth, 90
Paracelsus, 198–99
paranoia, 214
Parés, Oscar, 267–68
Parke-Davis pharmaceuticals, 56–57,
    56
PCP, 30–33
peripheral nervous system (PNS),
    2–3
Peru, 248–49, 257–58
Peterson, Jordan B., 90
peyote, *pl.18*, *39*, 261, 262–63
physical environment, 211
PiHKAL, 17, 69–70
Pinchot, Mary, 54–55
pleasure, 193
podcasts, 87–88, 230
Pollan, Michael, 90
Portugal, 252–53
post-traumatic stress disorder
    (PTSD), 119–25
preparation, 117
problematic use, 196
psilocin, 51–52
psilocybin, 33–37, 51–52
    about, 146–53
    adulterants and, 204
    depression and, 127–33
    research and, 78–79, 84–85
psychedelic-assisted psychotherapy,
    48–49, 57–58, *82*,
    116–19
psychedelic renaissance, 71–73
    ongoing research, 73–87
    rise of new industry, 93–97
    social and cultural contexts,
    87–93

psychedelics, 33–37. *See also* history; legal status; psychoactive substances
  brain level and, 100–101
  impact on brain function, 105–8, *106, 108*
  looking to the future, 217–24
  mental illness and, 112–15
  neuroreceptors and, 98–100
  psychological level and, 108–11
  resources, 225–33
Psychedelic Science 2023, 96–97
psychedelic societies, 227
psychoactive adulteration, 202
psychoactive substances. *See also specific substance*
  cannabinoids, 24–26
  depressants, 20–23
  dissociatives, 30–33
  empathogens/entactogens, 26–30
  explanation of, 12–14
  psychedelics, 33–37
  religious use, 260–61
  stimulants, 18–20
  types of, *pl.4,* 14–18
psychological level, 108–11
psychonauts and psychonautics, 14
psychopharmacology, meaning of, 13
psychosis, 209
psychotic reactions, 32, 35–36, 57
purity, 201–5

Ramstein, Susi, 41–42
rave culture, 235
Reagan, Ronald, 236
REBUS, 100–101
recovery position, 216

Reddit, 75–76
research
  addictions and, 134–40
  couples therapy, 142–43
  depression and anxiety and, 125–34
  looking to the future, 217–24
  microdosing, 143–45
  psychedelic, 73–87
  psychedelic-assisted psychotherapy, 116–19
  PTSD and, 119–25
  resources, 226–27
resources, 87–88, 225–33
resveratrol, 215
retreat centers, 97
Riba, Jordi, 77
Richards, William, 78–79
risks. *See also* harm reduction
  5-MeO-DMT, 167
  ayahuasca, 163–64
  cannabinoids, 24–26
  depressants, 21–23
  dissociatives, 31–33
  DMT, 163–64
  empathogens/entactogens, 28–30
  graph of, *pl.26, pl.27*
  ibogaine, 176–77
  ketamine, 190–91
  LSD, 157
  MDMA, 182–86
  mescaline, 172–73
  opioids, 23–24
  psilocybin, 152–53
  psychedelics, 34–37
  resources, 225–26
  stimulants, 19–20
Rogan, Joe, 90

Sabina, María, 51, *51*
Sacks, Oliver, 56
Sand, Nick, 55
Sandison, Ronald A., 44
Sandoz, 32–44, 52, 55, 61, 153
San Pedro, *pl.19*, 39–40
Sartre, Jean-Paul, 56
Saskatchewan Hospital, 45–47, *46*, 67
schizophrenia, 44–45, 209
screening, 117
self-knowledge, 193
sensory isolation tanks, *14*
sensory perceptions, 109, 149, 170
serotonin (5-HT), 5, *6–7*, 8
Sessa, Ben, 90
set and setting, *pl.13*, 32, 157, 190–91, 197–98, 208–13, *208*
shamanic cultures, 235
Shulgin, Alexander, 63–64, *64*, 69–70, *69*, 72, 264, *264*–66
Shulgin, Ann, 63–64, 69–70, *69*, 72, 264–66
Simon, Paul, 90
Single Convention on Narcotic Drugs, 236
smartphone apps, 230
Smith, Will, 90
smoking, 206
snorting, 206
Snyder, Derek, 16–17
socialization, 193
soft drugs, 15
Spain, 245–46, 249–51, 256, 262
Späth, Ernst, 40
spice, 25–26
Spring Grove Hospital, 57–58

SSRIs, 127
Stamets, Paul, 90
Stevens, Calvin, 56–57, 238
stimulants, 18–20
Sting, 90
St. John's wort, 207
Stolaroff, Myron J., 55–56, 69
Strassman, Rick, 77, 90
substitution, 202
Summer of Love, *60*
supplies, 211–12
surrender, 210
synapses, *pl.1*, 3–9, *4*
synesthesia, 109
synthesis-related impurities, 203

Thailand, 254
thin-layer chromatography (TLC), 205
Third Wave, The, 95–96
TiHKAL, 17, 70, 265
toad, 164–67
tolerance, 198–201
trafficking, 244–54
tramadol, 23–24
TripSit, 207
trip-sitting, 90–91
Tyson, Mike, 90

Unger, Sanford, *58*
United Nations Commission on Narcotic Drugs (CDN), 238
United Nations Convention on Psychotropic Substances, 62–63, *62*, 66
United States, 236–37, 241–43, 246–47, 259–60
Uruguay, 248–49

valerian, 207
vaporization, 206
Vietnam War, 59, 71
vital signs, 216
Vollenweider, Franz X., 77

war on drugs, 62–63, 72
Washington, 241–43
Washington, DC, 241–43
Wasson, Robert Gordon, 51–52, *51*
Wasson, Valentina, 51–52
Watts, Rosalind, 90

Wernicke-Korsakoff syndrome, 22
Wilson, Bill, 46–47
World Health Organization
    (WHO), 66, 187, 238

Yang, Andrew, 90
yohimbe, 207
YouTube channels, 229
yuppies, 95–96

Zeff, Leo, 64
Zinberg's Triangle, 197–98, *197*